Mothering, Mixed Families and Racialised Boundaries

T0347565

This pioneering volume draws together theoretical and empirical contributions analysing the experiences of white mothers in interracial families in Britain, Canada and the USA. The growth of the mixed race population reflects an increasingly racially and culturally heterogeneous society, shaped by powerful forces of globalisation and migration. Mixed family formations are becoming increasingly common through marriage, relationships and adoption, and there is also increasing social recognition of interracial families through the inclusion of mixed categories in census data and other official statistics. The changing demographic make-up of Britain and other western countries raises important questions about identity, belonging and the changing nature of family life. It also connects with theoretical and empirical discussions about the significance of 'race' in contemporary society.

In exploring mothering across racialised boundaries, this volume offers new insights and perspectives. The notion of racialisation is invoked to argue that, while the notion of race does not exist in any meaningful sense, it continues to operate as a social process. This crucial resource will appeal to academics, researchers, policy makers, practitioners and, undergraduate and post-graduate students.

This book was originally published as a special issue of *Ethnic and Racial Studies*.

Ravinder Barn is Professor of Social Policy at Royal Holloway, University of London, UK. She has published widely in the areas of 'race', ethnicity and children, and families.

Vicki Harman is Lecturer at Royal Holloway, University of London, UK. Drawing on her PhD research, she has written several papers about the situation of white mothers in mixed families.

Ethnic and Racial Studies
Series editors: Martin Bulmer, *University of Surrey, UK,* and
John Solomos, *City University London, UK*

The journal *Ethnic and Racial Studies* was founded in 1978 by John Stone to provide an international forum for high quality research on race, ethnicity, nationalism and ethnic conflict. At the time the study of race and ethnicity was still a relatively marginal sub-field of sociology, anthropology and political science. In the intervening period the journal has provided a space for the discussion of core theoretical issues, key developments and trends, and for the dissemination of the latest empirical research.

It is now the leading journal in its field and has helped to shape the development of scholarly research agendas. *Ethnic and Racial Studies* attracts submissions from scholars in a diverse range of countries, fields of scholarship and crosses disciplinary boundaries. It has moved from being a quarterly to being published monthly and it is now available in both printed and electronic form.

The *Ethnic and Racial Studies* book series contains a wide range of the journal's special issues. These special issues are an important contribution to the work of the journal, where leading social science academics bring together articles on specific themes and issues that are linked to the broad intellectual concerns of *Ethnic and Racial Studies*. The series editors work closely with the guest editors of the special issues to ensure that they meet the highest quality standards possible. Through publishing these special issues as a series of books, we hope to allow a wider audience of both scholars and students from across the social science disciplines to engage with the work of *Ethnic and Racial Studies*.

Titles in the series include:

**The Transnational Political
   Participation of Immigrants**
*Edited by Jean-Michel Lafleur and
   Marco Martiniello*

**Anthropology of Migration and
   Multiculturalism**
Edited by Steven Vertovec

Mothering, Mixed Families and Racialised Boundaries

Edited by

Ravinder Barn and Vicki Harman

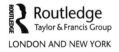

Routledge
Taylor & Francis Group

LONDON AND NEW YORK

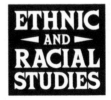

ETHNIC
◄ AND ►
RACIAL
STUDIES

First published 2014
by Routledge
2 Park Square, Milton Park, Abingdon, Oxfordshire OX14 4RN

and by Routledge
711 Third Avenue, New York, NY 10017, USA

First issued in paperback 2015

Routledge is an imprint of the Taylor & Francis Group, an informa business

British Library Cataloguing in Publication Data
A catalogue record for this book is available from the British Library

ISBN 13: 978-1-138-95369-7 (pbk)
ISBN 13: 978-0-415-73374-8 (hbk)

Typeset in Times New Roman
by Taylor & Francis Books

Publisher's Note
The publisher accepts responsibility for any inconsistencies that may have arisen during the conversion of this book from journal articles to book chapters, namely the possible inclusion of journal terminology.

Disclaimer
Every effort has been made to contact copyright holders for their permission to reprint material in this book. The publishers would be grateful to hear from any copyright holder who is not here acknowledged and will undertake to rectify any errors or omissions in future editions of this book.

Contents

Citation Information

The chapters in this book were originally published in *Ethnic and Racial Studies*, volume 36, issue 8 (August 2013). When citing this material, please use the original page numbering for each article, as follows:

Chapter 1
Mothering across racialized boundaries: introduction to the special issue
Ravinder Barn and Vicki Harman
Ethnic and Racial Studies, volume 36, issue 8 (August 2013)
pp. 1265–1272

Chapter 2
'Doing the right thing': transracial adoption in the USA
Ravinder Barn
Ethnic and Racial Studies, volume 36, issue 8 (August 2013)
pp. 1273–1291

Chapter 3
The experience of race in the lives of Jewish birth mothers of children from black/white interracial and inter-religious relationships: a Canadian perspective
Channa C. Verbian
Ethnic and Racial Studies, volume 36, issue 8 (August 2013)
pp. 1292–1310

Chapter 4
Researching white mothers of mixed-parentage children: the significance of investigating whiteness
Joanne Britton
Ethnic and Racial Studies, volume 36, issue 8 (August 2013)
pp. 1311–1322

Chapter 5

Social capital and the informal support networks of lone white mothers of mixed-parentage children
Vicki Harman
Ethnic and Racial Studies, volume 36, issue 8 (August 2013)
pp. 1323–1341

Chapter 6

Narratives from a Nottingham council estate: a story of white working-class mothers with mixed-race children
Lisa McKenzie
Ethnic and Racial Studies, volume 36, issue 8 (August 2013)
pp. 1342–1358

Please direct any queries you may have about the citations to clsuk.permissions@cengage.com

Notes on Contributors

Ravinder Barn is Professor of Social Policy in the Centre for Criminology and Sociology at Royal Holloway, University of London, UK.

Joanne Britton is Lecturer in Applied Sociology in the Department of Sociological Studies at Sheffield University, UK.

Vicki Harman is Lecturer in the Centre for Criminology and Sociology at Royal Holloway, University of London, UK.

Lisa McKenzie is a Research Fellow in the School of Education at the University of Nottingham, UK.

Channa C. Verbian currently works as a psychotherapist in private practice in Toronto, Canada.

Mothering across racialized boundaries: introduction

Ravinder Barn and Vicki Harman

Abstract

This introduction to the special issue 'Mothering across Racialized boundaries' begins by drawing attention to the symbolic importance of the inclusion of an interracial family in a sequence in the London 2012 Olympic opening ceremony. Following this, figures from the 2011 census in England and Wales are discussed in order to highlight increasing ethnic diversity and the growing number of people with mixed or multiple heritage. We consider the increasing social acceptance of interracial relationships as well as enduring stereotypes and critical questions asked of white mothers' parenting across racialized boundaries. We highlight the key themes from the literature relating to mothers in interracial families and introduce the papers featured in this volume.

Introduction

The opening ceremony of the London 2012 Summer Olympic Games directed by Danny Boyle portrayed an image of a confident multi-cultural Britain. It also incorporated a sequence devoted to popular music and culture from the 1960s to the twenty-first century. In this sequence a young black man, Frankie (Henrique Costa), and a young woman of mixed-parentage, June (Jasmine Breinburg), were shown to be falling in love as they travelled through a series of musical eras. The sequence also featured June's black father and white mother as well as other friends and family. Reflecting on this portrayal, Diane Abbott (2012), a British Labour Party politician, remarked on the symbolic importance of this scene:

> At no other point in Britain's history would an important ceremony like this revolve around a mixed-race family and a non-white young couple. And there is no other country in Europe that would have such a couple as symbolising youth in general. The high profile

given to this young couple shows how far Britain has come in its attitude to race.

Although most media accounts of the ceremony were indeed positive, the following day the *Daily Mail* published an article by Rick Dewsbury criticizing the portrayal of a happy middle-class interracial couple as 'politically correct' and 'absurdly unrealistic'. The article said that it must have been a 'challenge' for the organizers to find an 'educated white middle-aged mother and black father living together with a happy family in such a set up' (for further discussion, see Mix-d 2012). Commentators were quick to note that the Olympic Games features high-profile athletes from this very background, such as the British heptathlete Jessica Ennis, and the article was subsequently altered and then removed completely. This example reveals an interesting dynamic of a simultaneous normality and discomfort concerning ethnic diversity in general and in interracial families in particular. As well as drawing attention to the increasingly prominent portrayal of mixed families and relationships, it suggests that Britain still has a way to go before interracial families are accepted without reference to stereotypes in relation to lower-class status, lack of education or unhappiness.

Government statistics in Britain, Canada and the USA point to the increasing racial and cultural heterogeneity and the growth of the mixed-race population, reflecting wider processes of globalization and migration. At the same time, there is increasing social recognition of interracial families through the inclusion of mixed categories in census data and other official statistics. For example, the results of the 2011 census in England and Wales revealed that mixed/multiple-ethnic groups accounted for over one million people (2.2 per cent of the population). Of the pre-set mixed categories white and black Caribbean, white and Asian, white and black African and any other mixed, white and black Caribbean continued to be the largest. The growth of the mixed population can be located in a wider context where England and Wales is becoming increasingly ethnically diverse, with more people identifying with a minority ethnic group (ONS 2012). The 2011 census figures showed that the white British group has fallen from 87.5 per cent in 2001 to 80.5 per cent in 2011 (ONS 2012). The largest group following white British was any other white (4.4 per cent), which reflects an increase in people from Poland and other European countries in the last decade. Asian/Asian British (including Indian, Pakistani, Bangladeshi, Chinese and other Asian) accounted for 7.5 per cent of the population. Black/black British (which includes African, Caribbean and other Black) accounted for 3.3 per cent of the population of England and Wales. The census also showed considerable regional variation with London being the most ethnically diverse, with the highest proportions of minority ethnic groups and the lowest proportion of the white ethnic British group, at 44.9 per cent (ONS 2012). The changing demographic make-up of Britain and other western countries raises important questions about identity, belonging and the changing nature of family life. It also connects with theoretical and empirical discussions about the significance of race in contemporary society.

Although race has been discredited as an objective biological category, sociologists have drawn attention to the way that it has been difficult to lay to rest. Howard Winant (2006, p. 987), for example, argues that the concept of race 'persists, as idea, as practice, as identity, and as social structure'. One area where notions of race as well as ethnicity and identity continue to emerge is in relation to the social significance attached to mixed relationships and mixed or interracial families. Such family formations are becoming increasingly common through marriage, relationships and/or adoption. On one hand, the increasing number of interracial families can be seen to challenge notions of fixed, mutually exclusive groups with sharp distinctions between them (Hochschild and Weaver 2010). Such family relationships appear to illustrate the permeability and socially constructed nature of race. On the other hand, discussions of interracial families can sometimes imply that there are pure races that can be mixed or alternatively preserved. Similarly, the attention given to mixed relationships, including the concerns for the children that are sometimes articulated (e.g. will they have identity problems? Can they be happy?) can be seen to reify the notion of fixed and separate groups. Some writers have seen interracial relationships as a 'barometer' for relationships between minority and majority groups, suggesting that the greater social acceptance of minorities leads to more interracial relationships (Fryer 2007).

Within the academic literature, areas for exploration have included the visibility of interracial relationships in society (Okitikpi 2009) and the social construction of mixed race (Olumide 2002); the extent to which mixed-parentage and minority ethnic adopted children and interracial families experience racism (Tizard and Phoenix 2002; Okitikpi 2009; Harman 2010a; Barn and Kirton 2012); and the way in which such experiences are negotiated by white mothers (Banks 1996; Barn 1999; Harman 2010a; Caballero and Edwards 2010). Another key area for research has been the identity positions available to young people (Prevatt Goldstein 1999; Barn 2000; Tizard and Phoenix 2002; Barn and Harman 2006) and the way in which interracial identities are negotiated and/or transmitted within families and their wider support networks (Twine 2004; Tyler 2005; Caballero, Edwards and Puthussery 2008; Twine 2010). Furthermore, research has explored the nature and appropriateness of professional involvement in families' lives, with particular reference to social work (Banks 1996; Barn 1999, 2000; Okitikpi 2009; Harman 2010b). Scholarly work in this area has tended to focus primarily on the situation of children and in particular how they 'cope' with their mixed-ethnicity status or adjust in transracial adoptive family settings. In contrast, the experiences of white mothers of such children have traditionally received less attention, although arguably this is increasing. It has been noted that a critical gaze has been directed at white mothers of mixed-parentage children from sections of academic, media and professional audiences (Caballero and Edwards 2010). Given this, there is a need for a greater understanding of the experiences that mothers face in their day-to-day parenting.

This volume draws together theoretical and empirical contributions analysing the experiences of white mothers in interracial families in Britain, Canada and the USA. The collection of papers emerged out of a one-day conference titled 'Mothering across racialized boundaries', organized by the special issue editors at Royal Holloway, University of London in April 2010. Mothering was chosen as a particular focus for this special issue because although gender roles have changed considerably in western countries, much of the day-to-day parenting work continues to be done by women. Furthermore, white women have historically been seen as guardians of the 'purity' of the population (Ware 1992). As such, they have faced criticism and censure when involved in relationships with men from minority ethnic backgrounds, even though there is a growing discourse of ordinariness around mixed relationships (Caballero et al. 2012).

In exploring mothering across racialized boundaries, we invoke the notion of racialization (Miles 1989) to make it clear that while race does not exist in any meaningful sense, it continues to operate as a social process, or as Byrne (2006) illustrates in her study of mothers of young children in London, as a perceptual practice. We are interested in the social processes through which race becomes significant for interracial families, and the various papers presented here provide insights into the salience of this in Britain, Canada and the USA. Influenced by processes of migration and integration, the nature of racism and ethnic identities change over time, with implications for the context in which parenting takes place. It cannot be assumed that historical axes of discrimination will necessarily remain salient at the current time. Multiraciality has gained increased visibility with the election of Barack Obama as the first black president of the USA, and this has informed media and academic discussions (Jolivette 2012). We recognize that the experiences of interracial families are not static but dynamic and fluid, but we argue that it is important to listen for continuities as well as change.

The growth in research on minority parents' racial/cultural socialization practices has led to increased attention to how white parents in interracial families, particularly mothers, might engage in cultural competence practices (Vonk and Massatti 2008). Supporting the child to achieve cultural and racial competence is perceived as paramount, given the endurance of racism and colour discrimination in contemporary society. Parental attitudes and practices regarding racial and cultural identity, neighbourhood diversity and support networks are all held to be crucial in managing the tensions surrounding 'lived culture', essentialism and children's own preferences. Equally, the contrasting experiences of children and young people are an important area of focus and have received some consideration, particularly in the area of transracial adoption and interracial families (Samuels 2009).

In the first contribution to this volume, Ravinder Barn draws upon empirical research collated in New York to explore the complexities of transracial adoption and parenting. Located within the framework of racial and cultural socialization, the paper identifies three key perspectives to understand the ideology and practices of adoptive mothers: humanitarianism, ambivalence(ism), and transculturalism. It is argued that the ways in which white adoptive mothers understand and experience diversity and difference influences their approach to racial/ethnic socialization, which in turn is mediated through family and community networks and societal discourses on race, power and hierarchy.

In the second paper, Channa Verbian introduces the complex issues and experiences of racialization in the lives of white Jewish mothers of children from black/white interracial, inter-religious relationships. Using life history inquiry as an overarching research method, her paper is informed by her own personal history, literary narratives from three Jewish-American women and interviews conducted with two Jewish-Canadian mothers. This paper makes a valuable contribution in drawing attention to the salience of religion as well as race for socialization practices and identity.

Joanne Britton's article draws on the critical study of whiteness to emphasize the importance of examining white mothers' racialized identity and argues that an understanding of the sense of belonging of children and young people in mixed-parentage families can be enhanced by doing so. She also discusses kinship relationships and wider social networks as two related areas of investigation that can help to shed light on the nature of whiteness in mixed-parentage families.

Vicki Harman's paper contributes to a greater understanding of the support networks and social capital of lone white mothers of mixed-parentage children. She draws upon in-depth interviews with thirty mothers in Britain to analyse the range of informal support networks that mothers utilize in their parenting, including friends, family and support groups. Her findings suggest that close friendships between lone white mothers of mixed-parentage children were particularly valued for non-judgemental support and empathy, and it can be argued that such connections constitute a form of bonding capital. The paper also suggests that although racism impacted upon mothers' support networks, lone parenthood led to an impetus to enlarge their support networks by reaching out to individuals and organizations that they felt would be supportive of their parenting.

Finally, Lisa McKenzie's paper draws on findings from ethnographic research with thirty-five white mothers living on the St Ann's council estate in Nottingham, UK. The study examined how this group of women find value for themselves and their families in a context where outsiders often represent the estate and its residents as spaces and people of little value. The findings illustrate that mixing is highly valued because it offers status on the St Ann's estate and a chance to engage in a contemporary multicultural Britain.

Our interest in this special issue stems from the desire to examine the cultural and social contexts in which white mothers in interracial families negotiate parenting. Taken as a whole, the collection of papers draw attention to the importance of local/geographical, emotional and social locations, and highlights an increased emphasis on support networks and community relationships as well as the positive aspects of being in an interracial family. This volume also documents some continuities with regard to the critical questions and stereotypical assumptions that, at times and in some circumstances, continue to be directed at mothers who are parenting across racialized boundaries. The papers in this volume provide insight into areas for future investigation, including the need to find ways to include the voices of fathers in interracial families and document a range of methodological approaches that might usefully inform future research within this sensitive area of scholarship.

References

ABBOTT, DIANE 2012 'Race and the Olympics Opening Ceremony', *Jamaica Observer*, 5 August. [Available from: http://www.jamaicaobserver.com/columns/Race-and-the-Olympics-Opening-Ceremony_12152561 [Accessed 10 April 2013]]

BANKS, NICK 1996 'Young single white mothers with black children in therapy', *Clinical Child Psychology and Psychiatry*, vol. 1, no. 1, pp. 19–28

BARN, RAVINDER 1999 'White mothers, mixed-parentage children and child welfare', *British Journal of Social Work*, vol. 29, no. 2, pp. 269–84

——— 2000 'Race, ethnicity and transracial adoption', in Amal Treacher and Ilan Katz (eds), *The Dynamics of Adoption*, London: Jessica Kingsley Publishers

BARN, RAVINDER and HARMAN, VICKI 2006 'A contested identity: an exploration of the competing social and political discourse concerning the identification and positioning of young people of inter-racial parentage', *British Journal of Social Work*, vol. 36, no. 8, pp. 1308–24

BARN, RAVINDER and KIRTON, DEREK 2012 'Transracial adoption in Britain: politics, ideology and reality', *Adoption and Fostering*, vol. 36, no. 3, pp. 25–37

BYRNE, BRIDGET 2006 *White Lives: The Interplay of 'Race', Class and Gender in Everyday Life*, Abingdon: Routledge

CABALLERO, CHAMION and EDWARDS, ROSALIND 2010 *Lone Mothers of Mixed Racial and Ethnic Children: Then and Now*, London: Runnymede Trust

CABALLERO, CHAMION, EDWARDS, ROSALIND and PUTHUSSERY, SHUBY 2008 *Parenting 'Mixed' Children: Negotiating Difference and Belonging in Mixed Race, Ethnicity and Faith Families*, York: Joseph Rowntree Foundation

CABALLERO, CHAMION, *et al.* 2012 'The diversity and complexity of the everyday lives of mixed racial and ethnic families: implications for adoption and fostering practice and policy', *Adoption and Fostering*, vol. 36, no. 3, pp. 9–24

FRYER, ROLAND 2007 'Guess who's been coming to dinner? Trends in interracial marriage over the 20th century', *Journal of Economic Perspectives*, vol. 21, no. 2, pp. 71–90

HARMAN, VICKI 2010a 'Experiences of racism and the changing nature of white privilege among lone white mothers of mixed-parentage children in the UK', *Ethnic and Racial Studies*, vol. 33, no. 2, pp. 176–94

———— 2010b 'Social work practice and lone white mothers of mixed-parentage children', *British Journal of Social Work*, vol. 40, no. 2, pp. 391–406

HOCHSCHILD, JENNIFER and WEAVER, VESLA MAE 2010 'There's no one as Irish as Barack O'Bama': the policy and politics of American multiracialism', *Perspectives on Politics*, vol. 8, no. 3, pp. 737–59

JOLIVETTE, ANDREW 2012 *Obama and the Biracial Factor: The Battle for a New American Majority*, Bristol: The Policy Press

MILES, ROBERT 1989 *Racism*, London: Routledge

MIX-D 2012 *Museum Timeline 2012: London Olympics*. [Available form: http://www.mix-d. org/museum/timeline/london-2012-olympics [Accessed 10 April 2013]]

OKITIKPI, TOYIN 2009 *Understanding Interracial Relationships*, Lyme Regis: Russell House Publishing

OLUMIDE, JILL 2002 *Raiding the Gene Pool: The Social Construction of Mixed Race*, London: Pluto Press

ONS (OFFICE FOR NATIONAL STATISTICS) 2012 *Ethnicity and National Identity in England and Wales 2011*. Available from: http://www.ons.gov.uk/ons/dcp171776_290558.pdf [Accessed 10 April 2013]

PREVATT GOLDSTEIN, BEVERLEY 1999 'Black, with a white parent, a positive and achievable identity', *British Journal of Social Work*, vol. 29, no. 2, pp. 285–301

SAMUELS, GINA MIRANDA 2009 '"Being raised by white people": navigating racial difference among adopted multiracial adults', *Journal of Marriage and Family*, vol. 71, no. 1, pp. 80–94

TIZARD, BARBARA and PHOENIX, ANN 2002 *Black, White or Mixed Race? Race and Racism in the Lives of Young People of Mixed Parentage*, 2nd edn, London: Routledge

TWINE, FRANCE WINDDANCE 2004 'A white side of black Britain: the concept of racial literacy', *Ethnic and Racial Studies*, vol. 27, no. 6, pp. 878–907

———— 2010 *A White Side of Black Britain: Interracial Intimacy and Racial Literacy*, Durham, NC: Duke University Press

TYLER, KATHARINE 2005 'The genealogical imagination: the inheritance of interracial identities', *Sociological Review*, vol. 53, no. 3, pp. 476–94

VONK, ELIZABETH M. and MASSATTI, RICHARD R. 2008 'Factors related to transracial adoptive parents' levels of cultural competence', *Adoption Quarterly*, vol. 11, no. 3, pp. 204–26

WARE, VRON 1992 *Beyond the Pale: White Women, Racism and History*, London: Verso
WINANT, HOWARD 2006 'Race and racism: towards a global future', *Ethnic and Racial Studies*, vol. 29, no. 5, pp. 986–1003

'Doing the right thing': transracial adoption in the USA

Ravinder Barn

Abstract

Racial/cultural identity and parental cultural competence in transracial adoption (TRA) are subjects of fierce debate and discussion in contemporary western societies. The ongoing practice of TRA has led to a polarization that either supports or berates the suitability of the environment provided in such homes. The external scrutiny invariably creates doubt among white adoptive parents as to whether they are 'doing the right thing'. By drawing upon extant literature and original qualitative research carried out in New York, this paper explores adoptive mothers' conceptualization and understanding of racial/ethnic socialisation (RES). The paper puts forward three discursive approaches. It is argued that the ways in which white adoptive mothers understand and experience diversity influences their approach to RES, which in turn is mediated through family and community networks and societal discourses on race, power and hierarchy.

Background

Transracial adoption (TRA) is defined as an adoption that involves the placement of children in families that are racially and culturally different from them. In modern western societies, this practice largely involves the placement of minority ethnic children in white adoptive families.

International TRA in the USA began in the 1950s and 1960s with the adoption of Japanese and Korean children orphaned as a result of the Second World War and the Korean War (Weil 1984; Engel, Phillips and Dellacava 2007). The Vietnam War resulted in a further increase in TRA. With the emergence of international TRA, domestic TRA also became evident from the late 1950s involving the placement of Native American and later African American children. Indeed, this situation represents an astonishing juxtaposition involving the practice of domestic and international TRA alongside the then domestic anti-miscegenation laws preventing mixed marriages and relationships and therefore mixed families.

Significantly, in the 1960s, the beginning of TRA involving African American children was met with strong opposition. In 1972, the National Association of Black Social Workers (NABSW) called for an end to the practice of TRA, asserting that it constituted a form of 'cultural genocide'. Similar opposition from the Native American community led to the introduction of the Indian Child Welfare Act of 1978, which seeks to maintain Native American family life by allowing tribes exclusive jurisdiction in child welfare decisions including family placement. While no similar concessions were made to the African American community, it is estimated that the opposition to TRA from NABSW and other black-led groups and organizations resulted in a significant decline in such placements (Perry 1993–94).

In the 1980s and early 1990s, the domestic debate over TRA continued to persist; however, legislation was increasingly in support of TRA (Simon and Roorda 2007). In 1994, Congress passed the Multi-Ethnic Placement Act, which made it illegal for agencies to refuse to place a child with parents of another racial/cultural back-ground. Two years later, the 1996 amendment eliminated consideration of race altogether, making it a punishable offence that would result in the withdrawal of federal funds to agencies that emphasized race and culture in placement decision-making.

Arguably, four key factors led to a change in the legislation in support of TRA. These included the growing disproportionality of African American children in foster care, concerns about agencies' reluctance to place children with white families, an American-liberal stance to purge society of its racist past by placing TRA in the context of racial integration, and a critical mass of research evidence that claimed that such placements did no harm and were preferable to institutional care (Barth and Berry 1988; Shireman and Johnson 1988; Simon and Altstein 1996).

Today, however, another critical mass of research evidence points to the negative outcomes of TRA (both domestic and international) in terms of adverse effects on children's identity, belonging and culture (Andujo 1988; Hollingsworth 1997; Feigelman 2000; Samuels 2009; Vonk, Leea and Crolley-Simicb 2010; Zhang and Lee 2011). Con-versely, TRA also continues to be validated by other scholars who argue that the negative effects on identity are minimal or are outweighed by the benefits (Bartholet 2007; Simon and Roorda 2009).

While the research evidence base in the field of TRA remains contradictory and inconclusive with the polarized positions further entrenched, the practice of TRA continues to take place causing concern and controversy. Over the last forty years, almost half a million children from overseas have been adopted by parents in the USA (McGinnis et al. 2009). It is estimated that the vast majority of the adoptive parents are white and the adoptions are principally from Asian countries (mainly China and Korea), with the rest coming from Latin America, Eastern Europe and, most recently, Africa (Selman 2009). Domestic TRA rates, between 1995 and 2001, appear to have almost doubled for Hispanic children but have only marginally increased, from 14.2 per cent to 16.9 per cent, for African American children (Hansen and Simon 2004).

With the ongoing practice of TRA however, the twin themes of racial/cultural identity and parental cultural competence remain under scrutiny. However, it is important to point out that proponents and adversaries are agreed that TRA should be a last resort and that white adoptive parents must acquire the appropriate knowledge and skills to help children develop a positive racial/ethnic identity and the ability to navigate through the quagmire of a society preoccupied with race (Andujo 1988; Perry 1993–94; Simon and Altstein 1996; Hollingsworth 1997; Samuels 2009).

Theoretical framework

The notion of racial/ethnic socialization (RES) in TRA has emerged in the USA as an important theoretical framework to understand the processes at work in raising minority children to develop a healthy racial/ethnic identity and associated psychological well-being (Vonk 2001; Lee et al. 2006; Vonk et al. 2010). The process of socialization entails the acquisition of culturally relevant norms and values leading to successful adjustment and personal and social competence in children. This is said to occur through contextual learning via roles and in interaction with others. A key assumption is that parents play a crucial role in the racial and cultural competence of children. The primacy of the family as a key socializing agent suggests that TRA parents must themselves be culturally competent (Vonk 2001; Vonk and Massatti 2008).

It is now well recognized that minority parents play a vital role in educating their children about the structural and psychological implications of race as a social division in society (Lesane-Brown 2006). The concept of RES is considered to be complex and multi-dimensional, incorporating messages pertaining to racial identity, culture, inter-group interactions and discrimination. Studies into minority parenting practices have provided evidence of the requisite skills and knowledge in the processes of RES (Boykin and Toms 1985; Hughes and Chen 1999). From these, two key areas have been identified as significant:

1. *Cultural competence* – the transmission of cultural values, beliefs and behaviours that promote racial/ethnic identity development.
2. *Racial competence* – helping the child develop appropriate strategies to adequately confront prejudice, racism and discrimination.

The growth in research on minority parents' RES practices has led to increased attention into how white adoptive parents might engage in cultural competence practices (Vonk and Massatti 2008). Research from the 1980s suggested that white adoptive parents immersed the child primarily within the white environment and paid little or no attention to racial differences (McRoy et al. 1984; Andujo 1988). For example, in a study of sixty parents involved in trans-ethnic and same-ethnic placement of Mexican American children, Andujo (1988) reported that while same-ethnic families socialized their children with an emphasis on ethnicity, and taught racism survival skills emanating from their personal and social experiences, white adoptive parents de-emphasized ethnicity and adopted a largely colour-blind approach to socialization. Based on its findings of a 'potential ethnic identity formation problem for trans-ethnic adoptees', the study concluded that 'children wherever possible should be placed with parents of the same ethnicity or race' (Andujo 1988, p. 534). Although Andujo's findings appear to link the colour-blind socialization approach with white adoptive parents, it would seem that the key message is that the type of socialization approach employed is the crucial factor.

In their development of a cultural-racial identity model, Baden and Steward (2000) describe the conflicting challenge of identifying with both white parents' cultural group and one's own birth culture. In an earlier paper on the role of TRA parents, Baden and Steward (1997, p. 10) suggested that 'parental attitudes and beliefs that either affirm or discount the transracial adoptees' culture and racial group membership' would affect the development of cultural-racial identities.

In a study of parental attitudes towards birth culture, Scroggs and Heitfield (2001) report that while parents who had adopted from Asian countries attached greater importance to birth culture than those who had adopted from Eastern Europe, overall the children did not have close or frequent ties to people from their birth culture, which are considered important in generating a sense of affirmation and belonging to one's ethnic group. The authors argue that the majority of families in their study were not living in areas with high concentrations of people from the child's birth culture and that this may have prevented close, frequent ties. Similarly, in a quantitative study involving both domestic and international adoptive parents, Vonk et al. (2010) found that neighbourhood diversity and choosing child care providers from the child's ethnic background were a concern to fewer than half of their sample of 802 respondents.

As children grow older, adoptive parents' own interest and ongoing enthusiasm about RES have been found to diminish over time. In a study of African American adoptees in Minnesota, DeBerry, Scarr and Weinberg (1996) document that parents increasingly emphasised Eurocentric values and found that bicultural practices were not possible. Other studies focusing on international adoption have come to similar results. For example, Bergquist, Campbell and Unrau (2003) found that, over time, parents of Korean adoptees minimized or did not acknowledge the racial difference in their children and did not feel that their children were of a different race or ethnicity than themselves.

In a study of Chinese adoptees, Thomas and Tessler (2007) documented the importance of three key factors that had an important bearing in children's levels of Chinese cultural competence. These included parental attitudes towards bicultural socialization, parental social networks of Chinese adults, and the racial composition of the community. The presence of adults of the child's ethnicity within parents' friendship networks was highlighted as a key component associated with the above-mentioned three factors.

Much of the literature that has focused on adoptee's racial/cultural identity and parental socialization strategies makes an important contribution in raising our understanding of the crucial factors entailed in raising culturally and racially competent children. However, many of the existing studies into adoptive parents' RES practices, while important, fall short on three counts. First, they are primarily quantitative and lack the personal/authorial voice of adoptive parents. Second, many of the studies overlook the contested, complex and dynamic nature of RES. And finally, there is an under-theorization of the arguments.

Study aims/methods

This study aimed to build upon previous findings into RES practices in TRA. Qualitative in-depth semi-structured interviews were conducted with fifteen adoptive mothers in 2010, ranging in duration from sixty to ninety minutes. Since mothers are often perceived as the main transmitters of culture, and as many of the previous studies have included primarily mothers, it was decided in this study to only focus on their narratives (Johnston et al. 2007; Crolley-Simic and Vonk 2011). Perspectives of adoptive fathers are also important and should be studied in the future. Similarly, adoptee perspectives are crucial and may well contrast with those of parents (Samuels 2009). Only white adoptive mothers with children from a minority ethnic background were selected.

A minimum of four years together as a family was taken as a measure to obtain a sense of the efforts made by mothers to engage in RES practices and their own reflections on the successes and failures of their strategies. It was believed that given the previous concerns in the literature about the centrality of mixed neighbourhoods, a racially/ culturally diverse metropolis should form the backdrop for this study. The city of New York was therefore considered to be an ideal location in which to carry out this work.

The vast majority of the respondents who participated in this study lived in Manhattan, and two were resident in Brooklyn. All of the areas in which the participants were located were ethnically and racially diverse, although greater concentrations of some ethnic groups were found in a few localities. All respondents were recruited through snowball sampling. The inherent bias in such an approach needs to be recognized.

Profile of respondents

Given our focus on RES and the crucial significance of this in all TRA settings, both international (ten) and domestic (five) adoptions were included in this study. International adoptions involved children from China, Korea and South America. The majority of the domestic adoptions included African American/biracial children from New York.

With the exception of two mothers who had each adopted two children, the remainder of the sample had adopted one child only. The majority of the children were adopted as babies (eleven), four were adopted at the age of three, four, five and seven, and another two were adopted as teenagers. All except two of the children were female. Children's ages, at the time of study, ranged from seven to thirty.

The mothers in this study were well educated with a university education, and almost all were or had been in professional middle-class occupations. Mothers' ages ranged from forty-two to seventy-six, and the average age at the time of adoption was around forty-five. Mothers' occupations ranged from teachers, social workers, business analysts, and managers in health and social care institutions. The majority of the mothers (eleven) were married at the time of the study, as well as at the time of the adoption. The ethnic background of mothers recorded in the initial profile questionnaire included a range of self-definitions: Jewish (eight); white Anglo-Saxon Protestant (two); second-generation American (one); Caucasian (one); Italian American (one); white (two).

Data analysis

All interviews were recorded with the consent of the research participants and transcribed verbatim. A systematic analysis of the narratives was undertaken to analyse the qualitative data. This involved a process in which the theoretical framework of RES, discussed above, provided the structure within which to undertake the analysis.

Each interview was transcribed in full and subjected to a framework analysis. This included a five-stage approach including familiarization, identifying a thematic framework, indexing, charting and interpretation (Ritchie and Spencer 1994). The process included coding for an identification of themes; development of provisional categories and a relationship between these; and refinement of themes and categories against a backdrop of pre-existing knowledge and theory to develop new meanings and theory. Thus, a focus was placed on parental conceptualizations of race and ethnicity; attitudes and practices regarding the adopted child's birth culture; experiences of prejudice, discrimination and racism and parental efforts to fortify the adopted child against such negative experiences; parental and child networks; and racial and cultural diversity of the neighbourhood of adoptive families.

The thematic analytic framework helped to identify three discursive approaches discussed below (Edwards, Caballero and Puthussery 2010). It is recognized that there are inherent dangers of over-simplification and ambiguity in the employment of such categorization. Indeed, there is even overlap between categories as well as complexity within a category. It is important to note that such a framework was considered to be useful in understanding the accounts of the participants in this study.

In discussing the narratives of mothers, pseudonyms are used to preserve anonymity and confidentiality. Furthermore, in some cases actual names of the countries of origin have been disguised under a broad umbrella term to refer to a whole geographic region. For example, the continent name South America is employed in preference to individual countries to protect the identity of mothers and their adoptees.

Findings

The theoretical framework of RES and parental attributes/practices, discussed above, are employed to offer a discussion of the key findings. Arguably, these approaches represent discursive constructions of meaning about difference, belonging and identity as conceptualized by adoptive white parents in relation to their non-white adopted children (Schutz 1979). These approaches are identified by the author from the current study findings in the context of existing theory on RES and existing literature in this area.

The three approaches – humanitarianism, ambivalence(ism) and transculturalism – describe how parents in TRA seek to provide a sense of belonging and identity to their adopted children. At first, the difference between humanitarianism and ambivalence(ism) may appear to be rather minimal. While there may be some overlap between these approaches, they reveal racial and cultural nuances in white adoptive mothers' practices. The three discursive approaches are intended to provide a theoretical and empirical contribution to the TRA literature in the context of adoptive mothers' lived experiences. The findings below are presented as a polemic to invite debate and discussion.

Humanitarianism

The humanitarianism approach was found to be anchored within the love principle and entailed a de-emphasis upon race and ethnicity. Such an approach was common but not exclusive among those participants who had adopted internationally.

Humanitarianism conceptualizes race and ethnicity as insignificant and questions the notion of 'birth culture'. In the words of one white adoptive mother who had adopted from a Latin American country: 'She isn't culturally different...cos we got her as a new born...so she's part of our culture...Hispanics are not a race you know....'

Another mother who had adopted a biracial child from New York explained her sentiments about culture and history: 'Well, culture really doesn't come with you. Culture is kind of history...it's not your history...it's your birth family's history...the culture that they grew up in...you become part of the culture that you grow up in....'

Humanitarianism gives little significance to the need for friends and acquaintances that were from the adopted child's racial/cultural background. Such networks were not actively sought as the choice of friends was said to be not contingent upon individual ethnicities. Paradoxically, children's own friendship networks through school were described as racially diverse and perceived as a source of pride by the same parents.

Humanitarianism entails a de-emphasis upon race and ethnicity, viewing such considerations to be inconsequential: 'I mean I am kind of colour blind, I see her as a child in need of a parent, nothing more nothing less, I am a parent in need of a child, colour never came into it....'

Although they lived in one of the most racially and culturally diverse cities in the world, participants who embodied humanitarianism rcported that they had not actively attempted to immerse the child in their birth culture. This was largely due to a lack of perceived difference between themselves and their light-skinned Latin American or biracial child. One mother, who declared that she had not immersed her adopted child in her birth culture, reported a difficult encounter involving her adult adopted daughter, thereby raising the complex terrain of internal and external identity:

> There was a disconnect between who she was internally, to herself and who she was perceived to be [*pause*]...and it was a jolt I think, and she floundered [*pause*]...being perceived as a Hispanic meant nothing to her, it was a label put on her but that's not who she felt she was.

Racial and culture prejudice and discrimination were recognized as wrong. However, since the humanitarian view of their child was not based on racial structures in society, mothers responded in the fortification of their children with a reported love and understanding and in the emphasis of the beauty of their children's outward appearance:

> ...when she was at camp once the girls there called her a "flat face", and I said [*pause*] "your face is not flat, you've got a beautiful face, those girls probably called you that because they are jealous of you..." so I would try to ameliorate it like that...and I would say pay them no attention....

The humanitarian approach depicts a love of humanity and a disregard for racial difference and diversity. While this message is clear in the minds of the adoptive mothers themselves, it would appear that the external reality interferes with such thinking. Humanitarianism attempts to confront such challenges by focusing on the outward beauty of the adopted child, and by asking the external reality to recognize that the inner reality of the adopted child is different from their outward phenotype. Notably, many of the mothers in this group had adopted their children in the 1980s and 1990s. So it could be argued that such an approach resides in that era. The currency of such an approach in modern-day TRA is worthy of future research.

Ambivalence(ism)

Ambivalence(ism) was characterized by uncertainty and indecision about the adopted child's ethnic background and this was evident in mothers' discussions about their new interracial family formation.

For some of the participants, the skin tone of the child served as an important catalyst in their decision to adopt a minority child. It was evident that some mothers harboured a preference for light-skinned black children. This was tied up with feelings of ambivalence about race and ethnicity. One mother explained her preference for light skin: 'In my first assignment, I had fallen in love with a little boy who was 3 and half years old, and he was biracial . . . so I wanted this . . . he was not very dark . . . .'

Another mother also talked openly about the difficulties she had had in the early years in bonding with her adopted child due to the changes in his skin tone. Interestingly, the ambivalence for this mother was around whether she could raise a 'dark' male black child in contemporary American society, given her concerns about his future status as 'lowest on the rung':

> . . . in our society the darker you are the harder it is . . . and to be a black man is the hardest. You know you're the lowest on the rung. And I felt it was going to be more difficult for me, and for him, and also that he would be more acceptable if he was light.

The ambivalence of these women regarding race and ethnicity was reflected in their approach and practices as mothers. One mother of a seven-year-old internationally adopted Korean child conveyed her sense of hopelessness:

> I really don't know what to do with that difference [*pause*], I just don't know how to include [*pause*], how much to open that, I don't know anything about South Korea [*pause*], there was a Korean day parade and we took him and he wanted to leave, I don't know whether he is not ready [*pause*], or perhaps he sees that I don't know what to do with that piece of thing . . .

Unlike humanitarianism, the challenge of incorporating diversity into everyday life was palpable within ambivalence(ism) as mothers gave accounts of their efforts to embrace aspects of perceived difference, albeit invariably without success. In common with humanitarianism, the ambivalent approach also included mothers who reported that their children had a diverse set of friends; however, their own perceived ability to 'fit in' appeared to be an obstacle in forging racially/culturally diverse support networks. This seemed to be rooted in their concerns about their own ethnicity, socio-economic and/or adoptive status:

> . . . we took him to Tae Kwon Do in Queens, I thought it would be a community for me too so that I can have Korean mothers as friends, but everyone was not adoptive and I was the only white mother, I was entirely excluded by the mothers, and he [adoptive son] became like a show case, everybody was looking at him [*pause*], we went about 3 times and he didn't want to go again . . .

Although there were some efforts to connect with the child's racial/cultural heritage, the social networks of these mothers were reportedly devoid of adults who reflected the child's ethnic background. The racial and cultural heterogeneity of the neighbourhoods of New York and in some cases the schools attended by the children of these mothers however ensured that the children's friendship networks were diverse. One mother explained how her child seeks similarity and gravitates towards those who look like her: 'Last year, she came home and told us there is a girl in her class who is adopted from [South America]. I always think that she sees people who look like her.'

Another mother whose child attended a school where there were not many other children from the same background expressed regret that she had not made more of an effort towards the child's cultural heritage: 'I feel a little bit badly that I didn't push harder to teach her more about her [South American] heritage... but at the same time... she didn't really... evince a real interest... she became an American child right away....'

The theme of regret was not uncommon among mothers whose children were now young adults. Mothers talked about how they had never found the time to go to 'ethnic' restaurants related to the child's background, nor prepared food stemming from the child's birth culture.

Significantly, in their efforts to embrace the child's birth culture, mothers identified a number of obstacles ranging from the child's reported lack of interest, the incongruity between the adopted child and their 'ethnic' peers, and parents' self-reported lack of know-how on how to negotiate difference and diversity and feelings of discomfort and uncertainty.

The idea of equipping their adopted children with 'racial competence' was not one that had a particular resonance for these mothers. Many such mothers were unable to recall any incidents or acts of prejudice/racism directed at their children. Invariably, mothers described their child's negative experiences at school, among peers and so on as ones emanating from other factors such as the child's appearance, rather than in the context of their racial/ethnic difference. For example, one mother who reported struggling with her child's Asian identity explained: 'I don't think it's been directly about his race. This year, one boy was repeatedly picking on him... and he told him, "you have a big head".'

Transculturalism

A defining feature of transculturalism was an active cognizance of race and ethnicity. Mothers who embodied such an approach identified racism as pervasive, endemic and pernicious; and argued for a need to prepare adopted children for this reality. A focus on ethnicity and culture was regarded as part of such preparation.

The act of adoption for these women was imbued with cognizance, selflessness and altruism. The plight of children, whether as African Americans in the domestic foster care system or as orphans/unwanted children in their birth countries, was a key driver in these mothers' decision to adopt. Notably, the perceived disapproval of the anti-TRA lobby acted as a strong force to prove their cultural competence as mothers.

These mothers reported that they had intentionally chosen to live in predominantly African American and/or racially diverse communities so that their children could be among people who looked like them. Moreover, a distinction was drawn between segregated and integrated communities and networks. These mothers strived hard to ensure that there were adults in their networks who reflected the racial and cultural make-up of the adopted children. This involved extended family members, friends and social aunts and uncles from the neighbourhood. In addition, such efforts entailed finding babysitters, doctors, dentists and other professionals who looked like the child to act as role models. For some, such similarity was closer to home in their own wider network of family and friends:

> My husband's brother is married to a Korean woman; so I knew that a Chinese child in my family would not be the first and only person who would be Asian and who would have to deal with what this brings in our culture....

> My best friend is African American. Our neighbours, on either side of us are African American and West Indian . . . Umm Auntie Clara across the street has helped us with child care . . . both of the children have gone there before and after school . . . we make sure that some of the professionals we deal with are people of colour. We go to church, sometimes, with our next-door neighbour so that the kids are . . . you know . . . around with people that look like them . . . so we take it very seriously . . . .

Such networks were deemed important in helping adopted children with racial/ethnic identity development and reinforcement of positive messages, but also in equipping children to learn to deal with racism in society. One mother reported the importance of these support networks in helping her light-skinned biracial adopted daughter deal with self-image, and perceptions of others in racial/ethnic identification:

> . . . you know she would look in the mirror and see a white person. And Auntie Clara was also really helpful, you know, she would say, "you're black", "when society sees you they see a person of colour", "even white people may not know what you are, but most of them know you're not white".

Similarly, another mother talked about her social network and the importance of ensuring that there are adults from her child's ethnic background within this context. The role and influence of such individuals in the child's ethnic identity development was deemed crucial to provide a sense of nuanced complexity related to culture and belonging:

> ...and in ensuring that we have family and friends in our daily lives who are adult women who are Chinese American, who have come from China, or have always lived here, so that my daughter is not simply relying on me to refract for her on how an adult woman might make choices in relation to dealing with identity, but how women who are Chinese American make those choices every day...and my daughter would learn various different ways of experiencing Chinese heritage.

Transculturalism adheres to the diversity principle in such a way that it comes to be seen as an everyday reality for the racially mixed family. Mothers summed up the integral and embedded nature of their mixed family experience thus: 'You're never going to transcend race in the USA...maybe some day...she has partaken in our white culture and we have done that as well [taken part in black culture]...in a way... that feels intrinsic....'

These mothers emphasized the importance of birth culture in their children's lives. This often included various artefacts, books by authors from the child's ethnic background, music, dance and birth language classes. The active interest on the part of the mothers in such matters was clear. Moreover, such cultural socialization was not exclusive to the children's birth culture. One mother summed: 'From the very start, it was almost an inherent value that she would be raised in three cultures, Chinese, Jewish, and American. I had no other concept on how to raise her.'

In spite of her social networks that included Chinese adults, another mother of a Chinese adopted child talked about the challenges of integrating a Chinese heritage into the life of her child. It was believed that American society needed to make a greater effort to recognize the contributions of the Chinese American community. One way in which this could be done was said to be through schools. While individual adoptive parents made efforts to liaise with schools to encourage teachers to help include, for example, books by Chinese authors, music, dance and Mandarin lessons, it was believed that such changes could be made part and parcel of the school curriculum:

> I think there is an invisibility, there is much more of a consciousness around teaching African American heritage, which is for understandable reasons, the slave trade, the history of slavery, Jim Crow, racism up to today's daily cultural environment...but people from China have been here since the 1640s, so, there is quite a rich history, and we are in New York where there is enormous opportunity.

Interestingly, transculturalism revealed a complexity that recognized the importance of culture while demonstrating reflexive thinking based on personal experiences. For example, support networks such as Families with Children from China were described as invaluable; however, at the same time mothers demonstrated critical insight about the essentialism in cultural approaches. Mothers recognized that the celebration of Chinese holidays such as the New Year and the Moon Festival can be fun when the children are small but they may not be so exciting as the children grow older. Such changes were taken in their stride without undue worry and concern and showed self-assurance on the part of these mothers. One mother described the over-zealousness of some adoptive parents:

> I think sometimes they go a little over the top to keep their children connected to their culture . . . you know "Families with Children from China" is a nationwide thing . . . they publish a newsletter . . . .and there are recipes online on how to make moon cakes etc. I was telling Tammy's nanny about this, and she laughed and said, "nobody in China makes their own moon cakes, they go to the bakery" [*laughter*].

Discussion

While, within the social sciences, race is no longer seen as a biological entity but a social construction based on ancestry, skin colour and other phenotypic features, ethnicity has been defined as shared belongingness to a set of cultural attributes, language, religion, common geographic region and so on (Anthias and Yuval-Davis 1992). Such a framework can legitimately lead to a discourse that challenges ethnic boundaries to ask whether ethnicity is immutable and static.

The humanitarian approach, in this study, can be seen as posing a challenge to ethnic boundaries and the border guards at these racialized frontiers. The belief that a child's culture is not something they are born into but a culture in which they are raised confronts the notion of biology, blood and heritage (Patton 2000). In emphasizing love and understanding, the humanitarian approach seeks to inculcate belonging by minimizing difference. Several studies have noted that such minimization has been observed to increase over the lifetime of the adopted children as their interest in their birth culture declines (DeBerry et al. 1996; Bergquist et al. 2003). Furthermore, some evidence suggests that the more TRA parents are characterized as 'colour-blind', the less are their efforts towards cultural socialization for their children (Lee et al. 2006). In seeing children as the 'same' as yourself, or as American or as New Yorkers, it could be argued that the humanitarian approach rejects the ideology of difference and diversity and lays claim to the philosophy of humanity and the oneness of all irrespective of race and ethnicity. It may even be described as a post-race democratic cosmopolitanism. However, it is clear that the mothers in this study are engaged in a discursive discourse that is not necessarily challenging the existence of racialized boundaries of difference, but asserting the inclusion of the child within 'their' boundary as a way of instilling belonging.

This study shows that a humanitarian approach is characterized by a de-emphasis upon the adopted child's birth culture, especially if they are light-skinned and from a Latin American country (Andujo 1988). Indeed, in some cases phenotypic features and skin tone could be one explanation for a putative similarity with the adoptive mother's self-image and a de-emphasis on birth culture (Scroggs and Heitfield 2001). In other instances, for example within the ambivalent approach, it was evident that a child's biracial or multiracial ethnicity posed a significant challenge for the mothers. Indeed, these women's attitudes about race and ethnicity demonstrated an awareness of difference and diversity, but they questioned their own ability to deal with the 'race thing'. In comparison to humanitarianism and ambivalence(ism) approaches to children's race and ethnicity, the transcultural approach demonstrates an understanding of race and ethnicity that amalgamates mothers' experiences of their racially mixed families with a structural awareness of the pernicious effects of prejudice, discrimination and racism. Transculturalism embraces the integration of the intricacies of race and ethnicity into everyday life, demonstrates a cognizance of the transformational impact of becoming a mixed family, and claims support networks that are racially and culturally diverse (Thomas and Tessler 2007; Crolley-Simic and Vonk 2011; Twine 2010).

Research evidence into the experiences of TRA children shows that those who perceived their parents as supportive of RES reported higher levels of self-esteem compared with those who perceived their parents as unsupportive (Yoon 2004; McGinnis et al. 2009). Furthermore, transracial adoptee accounts suggest that parental de-emphasis of race signifies white 'parent's individual racial experience or world-view' and that adoptive parents have failed to see the world through their child's eyes (Samuels 2009, p. 92). This is said to result in situations where adoptive parents are emotionally unavailable when their children need them to navigate a highly racialised world (McGinnis et al. 2009).

In their study of parental attitudes towards birth culture, Scroggs and Heitfield (2001) suggest that the lack of racial and cultural heterogeneity of TRA families may have prevented close, frequent ties with adults from the child's birth culture. In this study, it is evident that families lived in a racially/culturally diverse metropolis and 'effort-making' to connect with the child's birth culture was arguably within the reach of most families. By exploring the evidence presented in this study, it is argued that parental attitudes towards race and ethnicity determined parental social networks. For some families, the presence of a diverse neighbourhood did not seem to afford opportunities in enhancing racial/cultural social capital (Putnam

2007). In the context of increasingly diverse but segregated communities, this is an important area for further study.

This finding is contrary to much of the previous literature that appears to present it as a given that a diverse neighbourhood has automatic inherent benefits in connecting transracial adoptees with their racial/cultural heritage (Feigelman 2000). Although it is recognized that a diverse community is likely to facilitate a child's network of friends via integrated schools and other social and community interactions, this study documents that parental efforts are crucial in making and sustaining diverse links in general and links with adults who reflect the child's ethnicity in particular.

Indeed, the TRA families in this study all met this key component outlined as crucial in much of the literature, that is, the importance of living in a racially/ethnically diverse neighbourhood. By looking at the discursive practices embedded within the transcultural approach, we can see that it is the awareness and understanding on the part of the parents and their attitudes and sensitivity towards race and ethnicity that result in particular relational and familial outcomes (Huh and Reid 2000; Yoon 2004). These include making efforts to embed themselves into the racial and ethnic fabric of the community and neighbourhood and to forge links with significant 'ethnic' adults within their own kinship, friendship and community networks. Furthermore, such mothers perceive the role and position of these adults as not peripheral but central to their everyday reality. Thus, mothers become active agents in ensuring that their adopted children are surrounded by diversity in a way that has meaning and significance.

This study recognizes that the ultimate aim of all mothers was for their children to be well adjusted and to feel at ease and comfortable with their self-image. However, the way in which mothers themselves perceived the child's ethnicity influenced their efforts to achieve cultural and racial competence in their children. While humanitarianism views the adopted children and parents as the same in cultural terms, ambivalence(ism) demonstrates some focus on cultural icons to enable the development of an ethnic identity and belonging. However, mothers who embodied the ambivalent approach reported being led by the children's enthusiasm and interest and conveyed a passive approach to racial/cultural socialization (Samuels 2009). Transculturalism, on the other hand, shows a portrayal of mothers as active agents who embraced and embedded diversity into their lives in a way that it was not just the child who was in need of cultural and racial competence, but that they themselves as an interracial family needed to grow together. Hence, the addition of key individuals into their familial and social network, and the importance of challenging wider structures to bring about greater understanding and awareness were regarded as crucial (Vonk 2001).

Conclusion

The findings of the present study are based on a limited sample of white adoptive mothers and thus caution is needed in the interpretation and application of these results for wider applicability. Nevertheless, the rich and honest accounts of the study participants reveal important insights into 'lived culture', essentialism and dealing with children's own 'preferences'. By documenting empirical findings and extant literature, the paper offers a theoretical framework to explore intersections between, for example, parental perspectives and neighbourhood diversity.

In an exploration of the narratives of white adoptive mothers, this study shows that parental conceptualizations of race and ethnicity are an important determinant in mothers' world view. This has an impact on their construction of family and community networks, which in turn influences the child's notion and understanding of belonging and culture. While humanitarianism, in minimizing racial/cultural difference, may be a challenge to the socially constructed racialized boundaries, it nonetheless may obscure the realities of power differentials and could prevent the development of children's cultural and racial competence in a society that continues to be preoccupied with race. The ambivalence(ism) approach shows that mothers' own identity development in a racially/culturally mixed family may be in a state of flux in the context of the dynamic and fluid nature of culture, identity and belonging. Parental transference of ambivalence towards belonging and identity may result in similar practices to those of humanitarianism. The transculturalism approach provides important insights into mothers' strategies to inculcate cultural and racial competence in children. The approach resembles more closely the ascribed racial and cultural socialization embedded within the cultural competence framework. However, there is a danger of reification of race and culture in the uncritical embracement of such an approach. Moreover, it is evident from the accounts of mothers that neighbourhood diversity in and of itself is insufficient in developing and maintaining social networks, but that parental efforts to seek and nurture appropriate social relationships can add to their and their child's overall experience and contribute to identity, belongingness and culture.

References

ANDUJO, ESTELA 1988 'Ethnic identity of transethnically adopted Hispanic adolescents', *Social Work*, vol. 33, no. 6, pp. 531–5

ANTHIAS, FLOYA and YUVAL-DAVIS, NIRA 1992 *Racialised Boundaries: Race, Nation, Gender, Colour and Class and the Anti-Racist Struggle*, London: Routledge

BADEN, AMANDA L. and STEWARD, ROBBIE J. 1997. '*The role of parents and family in the psychological adjustment of transracial adoptees: Implications for the Cultural-Racial*

Identity Model for transracial adoptees'. Paper presented at the meeting of the Fourteenth Annual Teachers College Roundtable on Cross-Cultural Psychology and Education.

BADEN, AMANDA L. and STEWARD, ROBBIE J. 2000 'A framework for use with racially and culturally integrated families: the cultural-racial identity model as applied to trans-racial adoption', *Journal of Social Distress and Homelessness*, vol. 9, no. 4, pp. 309–37

BARTH, RICHARD and BERRY, MARIANNE 1988 *Adoption and Disruption*, New York: Aldine de Gruyter

BARTHOLET, ELIZABETH 2007 'International adoption: thoughts on the human rights issue', *Buffalo Human Rights Law Review*, vol. 13, pp. 151–98

BERGQUIST, KATHLEEN, CAMPBELL, MARY E. and UNRAU, YVONNE A. 2003 'Caucasian parents and Korean adoptees: a survey of parents' perceptions', *Adoption Quarterly*, vol. 6, no. 4, pp. 41–58

BOYKIN, A. WADE and TOMS, FORREST D. 1985 'Black child socialization: a conceptual framework', in Harriette Pipes McAdoo and John Lewis McAdoo (eds), *Black children: Social, educational, and parental environments*, Thousand Oaks, CA: Sage Publications

CROLLEY-SIMIC, JOSIE and VONK, ELIZABETH M. 2011 'White international transracial adoptive mothers' reflections on race', *Child and Family Social Work*, vol. 16, no. 2, pp. 169–78

DEBERRY, KIMBERLEY M., SCARR, SANDRA and WEINBERG, RICHARD 1996 'Family racial socialisation and ecological competence: longitudinal assessments of African-American transracial adoptees', *Child Development*, vol. 67, no. 5, pp. 2375–99

EDWARDS, ROSALIND, CABALLERO, CHAMION and PUTHUSSERY, SHUBY 2010 'Parenting children from "mixed" racial, ethnic and faith backgrounds: typifications of difference and belonging', *Ethnic and Racial Studies*, vol. 33, no. 6, pp. 949–67

ENGEL, MADELINE, PHILLIPS, NORMA K. and DELLACAVA, FRANCES A. 2007 'International adoption: a sociological account of the US experience', *International Journal of Sociology and Social Policy*, vol. 27, no. 5/6, pp. 257–70

FEIGELMAN, WILLIAM 2000 'Adjustments of transracially and inracially adopted young adults', *Child and Adolescent Social Work*, vol. 17, no. 3, pp. 165–83

HANSEN, MARY ESCHELBACH and SIMON, RITA J. 2004 'Transracial placement in adoptions with public agency involvement: what can we learn from the AFCARS data?', *Adoption Quarterly*, vol. 8, no. 2, pp. 45–56

HOLLINGSWORTH, LESLIE DOTY 1997 'Symbolic interactionism, African-American families, and the transracial adoption controversy', *Social Work*, vol. 44, no. 5, pp. 443–53

HUGHES, DIANE and CHEN, LISA 1999 'The nature of parents' race-related communications to children: a developmental perspective', in Lawrence Balter and Catherine S. TamisLemonda (eds), *Child Psychology: A Handbook of Contemporary Issues*, New York: Psychology Press

HUH, NAM SOON and REID, WILLIAM J. 2000 'Intercountry, transracial adoption and ethnic identity: a Korean example', *International Social Work*, vol. 43, no. 1, pp. 75–87

JOHNSTON, KRISTEN E. *et al.* 2007 'Mothers' racial, ethnic, and cultural socialization of transracially adopted Asian children', *Family Relations*, vol. 56, no. 4, pp. 390–402

LEE, RICHARD M. *et al.* 2006 'Cultural socialization in families with internationally adopted children', *Journal of Family Psychology*, vol. 20, no. 4, pp. 571–80

LESANE-BROWN, CHASE L. 2006 'A review of race socialization within black families', *Development Review*, vol. 26, no. 4, pp. 400–26

MCGINNIS, HOLLEE *et al.* 2009 *Beyond Culture Camp: Promoting Healthy Identity Formation in Adoption*, New York: Evan B. Donaldson Adoption Institute

MCROY, RUTH G, ZURCHER, LOUIS, A and LAUDERDALE, MICHAEL L. 1984 'The identity of transracial adoptees', *Social Casework*, vol. 65, no. 1, pp. 34–9

PATTON, SANDRA 2000 *Birth Marks: Transracial Adoption in Contemporary America*, New York: New York University Press

PERRY, TWILA L. 1993–94 'The transracial adoption controversy: an analysis of discourse and subordination', *New York University Review of Law and Social Change*, vol. 21, no. 3, pp. 33–107

PUTNAM, ROBERT D. 2007 'E pluribus unum: diversity and community in the twenty-first century: the 2006 Johan Skytte Prize Lecture', *Scandinavian Political Studies*, vol. 30, no. 2, pp. 137–74

RITCHIE, JANE and SPENCER, LIZ 1994 'Qualitative data analysis for applied policy research', in Alan Bryman and Robert G. Burgess (eds), *Analysing Qualitative Data*, London: Routledge, pp. 173–94

SAMUELS, GINA MIRANDA 2009 '"Being raised by white people": navigating racial difference among adopted multiracial adults', *Journal of Marriage and Family*, vol. 71, no. 1, pp. 80–94

SCHUTZ, ALFRED 1979 'Concept and theory formation in the social sciences', in John Bynner and Keith Stribley (eds), *Social Research: Principles and Procedures*, London: Longman [first published in 1954], pp. 44–66

SCROGGS, PATRICIA and HEITFIELD, HEATHER 2001 'International adopters and their children: birth culture ties', *Gender Issues*, vol. 19, no. 4, pp. 3–30

SELMAN, PETER 2009 'The rise and fall of intercountry adoption in the 21st century', *International Social Work*, vol. 52, no. 5, pp. 575–94

SHIREMAN, JOAN and JOHNSON, PENNY 1988 *Growing up Adopted*, Chicago, IL: Chicago Child Care Society

SIMON, RITA J. and ALTSTEIN, HOWARD 1996 'The case for transracial adoption', *Children and Youth Services Review*, vol. 18, nos. 1–2, pp. 5–22

SIMON, RITA J. and ROORDA, RHONDA M. 2007 *In their Parents' Voices*, New York: Columbia University Press

SIMON, RITA J. and ROORDA, RHONDA M. 2009 *In Their Siblings' Voices : White Non-Adopted Siblings Talk about Their Experiences Being Raised with Black and Biracial Brothers and Sisters*, New York: Columbia University Press

THOMAS, KRISTY A. and TESSLER, RICHARD C. 2007 'Bicultural socialisation among adoptive families: where there is a will, there is a way', *Journal of Family Issues*, vol. 28, no. 9, pp. 1189–219

TWINE, FRANCE WINDDANCE 2010 *A White Side of Black Britain: Interracial Intimacy and Racial Literacy*, Durham, NC: Duke University Press

VONK, ELIZABETH M. 2001 'Cultural competence for transracial adoptive parents', *Social Work*, vol. 46, no. 3, pp. 246–55

VONK, ELIZABETH M., LEEA, JAEGOO and CROLLEY-SIMICB, JOSIE 2010 'Cultural socialization practices in domestic and international transracial adoption', *Adoption Quarterly*, vol. 13, nos. 3–4, pp. 227–47

VONK, ELIZABETH M. and MASSATTI, RICHARD R. 2008 'Factors related to transracial adoptive parents' levels of cultural competence', *Adoption Quarterly*, vol. 11, no. 3, pp. 204–26

YOON, DONG PIL 2004 'Intercountry adoption: the importance of ethnic socialization and subjective well-being for Korean-born adopted children', *Journal of Ethnic and Cultural Diversity in Social Work*, vol. 13, no. 2, pp. 71–89

WEIL, RICHARD H. 1984 'International adoption: the quiet migration', *International Migration Review*, vol. 18, no. 2, pp. 276–93

ZHANG, YUANTING and LEE, GARY R. 2011 'Intercountry versus transracial adoption: analysis of adoptive parents' motivations and preferences in adoption', *Journal of Family Issues*, vol. 32, no. 1, pp. 75–98

The experience of race in the lives of Jewish birth mothers of children from black/white interracial and inter-religious relationships: a Canadian perspective

Channa C. Verbian

Abstract

In this paper, I discuss my life history study on experiences of race in the lives of Jewish-Canadian and Jewish-American birth mothers of children from black/white interracial, inter-religious relationships. Opening with a reflection on my personal experience and what compelled me to undertake this research, I then provide a short introduction to attitudes about interracial/inter-religious relationships found in the literature, followed by an introduction to my research methodology. Finally, I compare and contrast the experiences of three Jewish-American mothers, excerpted from their published narratives, and the experiences of two Jewish-Canadian mothers from two recorded interviews, with my own experience. I conclude this paper with a brief summary of the emerging themes in my research and how they add to our understanding of mothering across racialized boundaries.

Background

As a Jewish-Canadian mother of children from a black/white interracial, inter-religious relationship, I wanted to be proactive about my children's social and psychological development. Consulting the literature on interracial children and racial-identity formation, I became increasingly curious about the experiences of white mothers and how everyday racism and racial discourses might affect their social and psychological well-being. When my subsequent search for literature on racially or religiously heterogeneous mother/child relationships yielded few results (Verbian 2006), I became inspired to investigate how white Canadian mothers of children from interracial unions experience race for my doctoral research.[1] The rationale for this paper, which focuses specifically on Jewish mothers of black/white interracial children, began while interviewing my participants. As my interviews proceeded, I recognized that although I am phenotypicaly white, aspects of my experience differed from the non-Jewish mothers. Frankenberg (1993) illuminates this difference stating that non-Jews often view Jews as racial 'Others', hence Jewish (women's) identity is articulated not only in terms of engagement with (or disinterest in) a cultural form, but also as recognition of belonging to a group that faced, and still faces, discrimination and violence. In this way, Jewish women, like black women, are racialized as non-white. Elaborating, Brodkin (1998) states that [America] both 'assigns Jews to the white race' and 'creates an off-white race for Jews to inhabit'. My experience, growing up Jewish in Canada's Christian cultural hegemony, often reflected these findings. While reasons for 'racialized othering'[2] are beyond this paper's scope, the following summary provides an overview of attitudes towards interracial and inter-religious relationships.

Published more than two decades ago, Spickard's (1989) comprehensive study of interracial and inter-religious marriage and ethnic identity in twentieth-century America provides a well-documented overview of opposition to intermarriage. According to Spickard (1989), while reactions have varied depending on time, place, social class, gender and a union's formality, the white population's 'near hysterical' disapproval has been consistent, even after the abolishment of the last anti-miscegenation laws in 1967 (Spickard 1989, p. 283). Winks (1997) in his definitive history of Canada's black population, states that Canadian law, like British law, did not prohibit interracial marriage between blacks and whites. While I could not find current literature on interracial marriage in Canada, popular press articles showcasing interracial unions do suggest that racism and racialization affect these couples (*Globe and Mail*, 3 April 2008, L2; *Toronto Star*, 11 March 2000, K1). In Britain, Harman's (2010) research on lone white mothers of mixed-race children, and Tizard and Phoenix's (2002) research on race and racism in the lives of British youth of mixed parentage, also suggests disapproval of interracial relationships. Acknowledging that literature problematizing interracial relationships is common, Edwards et al. (2012, p. 1) also identify research viewing interracial relationships as ordinary, unremarkable features of today's multicultural social life. While it is difficult to ascertain the level of acceptance, increased attention to interracial relationships is evident.

According to some who study interracial families, in the last three decades black/white interracial heterosexual relationships, including marriage and cohabitation, has increased in the USA (Spickard 1989; Zack 1995; Root 1996; Hill and Thomas 2000), Britain (Barn 1999; Goldstein 1999; Tizard and Phoenix 2002; Winddance Twine 2004) and Australia (Luke and Luke 1999). In Canada, Hill's (2001) autobiography about growing up with interracial parents in Toronto and a prominent newspaper series profiling 'multiracialism' (Infantry 2000) have received attention. More recently, Toronto's *Globe and Mail* (2008) newspaper highlighted Canadian census data indicating that the number of individuals in interracial relationships rose from 2.6 per cent in 2001 to four per cent in 2006. Of these nearly 300,000 individuals, 47,105 were black with a white partner. Although statistically the number of interracial relationships is relatively low, they point to a trend.[3] Statistics gathered in 2001 on Jewish heterosexual inter-religious marriage show 54 per cent of the marriages of self-identified American Jews and 25–30 per cent of self-identified Canadian Jews as inter-religious (DellaPergola 2009). While there are no Canadian statistics on Jewish/black unions, American studies suggest that Jews form the second-largest group to intermarry with a black partner (Senna 2004). Gibel Azoulay (1997), an observant Jew and African studies scholar with a Jewish mother and a black father, questions the attention paid to relationships between blacks and Jews in the USA. I believe this attention results, in part, from the aftermath[4] of shared involvement in the American civil rights movement. Canada's black and Jewish populations have no similar history.

My interest in Jewish women's experiences of race is partially motivated by my own experience. As a Jewish woman who had experienced anti-Semitism, I felt written out of the research on raising interracial children. Reading both Greene (1990) and Collins (1994), I was surprised at how they juxtaposed black and white maternal experience and seemed to suggest the necessity of privileging an interracial child's black identity in order to mitigate experiences of anti-black racism. According to Greene (1990, p. 208) a 'Black mother's role in raising children is accompanied by tasks not shared by their White counterparts, specifically racial socialization of Black children.' Collins (1994, p. 57) elucidates this idea further:

> Motherhood occurs in specific historical contexts framed by interlocking structures of race, class and gender, a context where the sons of White mothers "have every opportunity and protection", and the "colored" daughters and sons of racial ethnic mothers "know not their fate".

McKenzie's (2009) research on the intersection of race, class and gender in the lives of single white mothers of interracial children living in a British council estate presents an alternative view.

I believe Greene (1990) and Collins' (1994) focus on a child's paternal identity racializes and essentializes maternal experience, and de-emphasizes the importance of the maternal bond. In the context of Jewish life, according to the *Mishnah* (redacted circa 220 CE), the oldest codified normative definition used by Jews for self-identification, the transmission of Jewish identity is matrilineal. To privilege the black paternal identity of a Jewish woman's child seems to render her cultural heritage invisible.

My children's father, believing that our children would experience anti-black racism and anti-Semitism, encouraged them to acknowledge and embrace both identities. Now in their late twenties, they identify as Jewish by faith and both black and Jewish culturally. Light skinned and interested in western art and culture, their black peers often denigrate them as being too 'white' or too 'Jewish'. Jewish peers, often fascinated by their mixed heritage, have difficulty understanding how they embrace a mixed identity. Speaking with ease, my children assure me that I am not their 'racial other'. In this way, my experience differs from the literature where interracial children commonly feel their mothers cannot understand. Lazarre (1996) writes about her son's words with sadness. I am curious if Lazarre speaks to him about anti-Semitism as I do with mine, and if it is this that shelters us from a racial divide.

Reflecting, my daughter's birth in 1983 marks the beginning of my informal research on racialized mothering. Unconcerned about crossing social boundaries, I was surprised when I was frequently asked: 'What about your child?' Outwardly, unwavering, I said I did not share their worry. Inwardly, I asked myself why does this question feel shaming. As time passed, and others' questions changed to whether my children were being raised 'black' or 'Jewish', so too, did mine. No longer focused on how to raise interracial, inter-religious children, I became curious about how racializing attitudes may affect white mothers of interracial children.

Methodology

As stated above, the initial motivation for my research was my subjective interest in how my experience of race mirrored and differed from other white mothers with interracial children. Because of this, I chose a methodology that encourages reflexivity. According to Caughey (2006), life history recognizes and emphasizes the important influence of 'multiple cultural traditions' on an individual's life, allowing the researcher to compare and contrast their own social and cultural orientation with that of their co-researchers. Further, as Cole and Knowles (2001, p. 11) assert, life history inquiry is about 'gaining insights into the broader human condition by coming to know and understand the experiences of other humans...how individuals walk, talk, live, and work within [their] particular context.' Using focused inquiry during my two, two-hour long, recorded semi-structured conversations with my co-researchers provided me with rich narrative data about the meaning and experience of race in these mothers' lives.

Complementing the life history methodology, I integrate aspects of arts-informed research. Cole and Knowles (2008) describe arts-informed research as an inclusive approach to both the inquiry process and representation that honours diverse forms of knowing about the everyday experience of research participants. To 'know' the experience of the Jewish and white mothers in my study, my data are comprised of both the recorded narratives from my interviews and the literary narratives of the American woman. Luke and Luke (1999, p. 246) discuss narrativization's specific value for expessing personal stories related to race:

> People's narrativizations in the interview context of their histories, experiences, and interpretations – are the only texts available to us with which to investigate and understand how dominant discourses on race mesh with people's sense-making and blending of cultural values and practices, and how racializing practices are experienced, reinterpreted, and retold.

Narrativization helped me to both hear and portray the poignancy of these mothers' stories, something that a more traditional methodology may not have captured.

Findings

The findings I present are excerpted from my doctoral research on the experience of race in the lives of white birth mothers of children from black/white interracial relationships. Focused on Jewish women, they are not meant to be complete, comprehensive or conclusive; rather, they introduce racialized experience in my life, in the published narratives of three Jewish-American mothers, Ruth McBride Jordan, Jane Lazarre and Hettie Jones, and in the narratives of the two Jewish-Canadian mothers I interviewed in 2010. Given the life history and arts-informed research methodologies I employed, my findings are presented with a deliberately narrative quality.

Although the narratives of Jordan, Lazarre, Jones and myself begin in New York City, my narrative moves to Toronto. Because of this, I believe that aspects of our experiences differ. Canadian federal policy emphasizes multiculturalism and the retention of one's ethnic and cultural identity, unlike the American melting pot, which emphasizes a unified American identity in spite of its racial divide (AECMMT 1995). While Canada shares collective guilt for racist and colonial practices that built our nation, Canada does not share America's collective guilt for the mass enslavement of Africans and the subsequent legalized segregation that prevailed well into the twentieth century (Winks 1997). Although Jordan, Lazarre, Jones and I share Jewish roots, our experience with anti-black racism differs. An analysis of how these differences affect our maternal identity is beyond the scope of this paper. Even still, born in different decades and different countries, there are parallels in our experience.

James McBride's mother,[5] Ruth McBride Jordan, born in 1921 in Poland to a Rabbi and his wife, emigrated to the USA at two years old; first to New York and then to Virginia. Jordan was exposed to southern black culture early in life, helping out in her family's small general store that served black customers in the segregated South. Her life was harsh. Her family struggled financially and lived in fear of anti-Semitism and the Ku Klux Klan. At home, with her mother suffering ill health and partial post-polio paralysis, her father sexually abused her; at school, her white Christian classmates ostracized her. Lonely, she secretly befriended a young black man with whom she became pregnant at the age of fifteen. Her mother, believing that Jordan was at risk of being killed by the Ku Klux Klan, if not by her father, advised her to visit her grandmother in New York where an illegal abortion could be arranged. This visit opened Jordan to alternatives outside of her oppressive life in Virginia. At seventeen, after graduating from high school, Jordan moved to her grandmother's in New York to work in her aunt's leather factory. Here, in 1939, she met her aunt's 'best worker', Andrew Dennis McBride, who took her under his wing. Soon the naive Jordan, 'drawn to the fast life', quit her job and moved to Harlem were she became the target of a pimp. Scared and missing her mother, she called McBride who convinced Jordan to return to her grandmother. Before long, this unlikely couple married, with McBride, a kind and gentle, stridently religious black Baptist man, providing her with the first stability she had known. Adopting her husband's life, Jordan left her birth family, distanced herself from her Jewish identity, changed her Jewish name, and became Baptist. At age thirty-six, sixteen years and eight children later, Jordan lost McBride to cancer. She married Hunter Jordan, with whom she had another four children. In 1972, Jordan was tragically widowed again.

Although painful, American author Hettie Jones's (born Cohen in 1934),[6] story is less tragic than Jordan's. Living in a lower middle-class neighbourhood in Queens, New York, Jones grew up in a family keen to be Americans. They never spoke about their Eastern European origins, kept kosher laws loosely, and spoke Yiddish, the language of Ashkenazi Jewry, only to hide something from their children. Still, Jones remembers getting the impression from her family that she should not mix with the few neighborhood 'Anglos' and 'Irish', except when unavoidable. Her father was a blue-collar worker in Manhattan; her mother, a homemaker, actively volunteered for Jewish organizations. Jones remembers her mother humming as they ironed linen together, enjoying women's magazines, and putting on mink and amethysts before treating herself to a Broadway play. Of her dad she writes: 'We were joined at the heart, not at the head' (Jones 1990, p. 8). Once, finding Jones reading 'one of the two books' in their home, he exclaimed, 'you won't find life there' (Jones 1990, p. 8). This suburban life her parents coveted was not the life for her. She wanted 'something different'. To this end, in high school, she played atonal music and 'hung out' with boys who spoke about anarchy. After her undergraduate drama studies, she attended graduate school at New York's Columbia University. Later, Jones settled into the burgeoning bohemian life of Greenwich Village in the 1950s and 1960s, working at the *Record Changer*, a magazine for collectors of jazz. Here she met the yet-to-be-published poet, Leroi Jones,[7] who she describes as patient and intelligent with roots 'more middle-class' than her own. Soon, in love and pregnant with the first of their two daughters, Jones, risking all connection with family, entered a marriage that would not last. While it would seem simplistic to say that being white and Jewish caused their marriage to fail, on reading Jones's memoir (1990), we see this played a significant part. For her husband, who became part of the vanguard of the Black Power movement, marriage to a white and Jewish woman became untenable.

Of these three women, Jane Lazarre (1976, 1996),[8] who grew up in a progressive New York Jewish intellectual family in the 1950s, was the only one raised to embrace notions of racial equality, 'colour-blindness', social justice and diversity. Still, the only black people she interacted with were her family's domestic workers who cleaned or cared for the children. Lazarre writes of her teenage years as lonely and troubled, the consequence of her mother dying when Lazarre was seven. Her college years changed this when she found meaning through involvement in the American civil rights, labour and women's movements. She met her husband in 1966 while picketing the welfare offices where she worked. True to his values, Lazarre's father accepted him, referring to him as the 'strong and reliable Negro chap who married his often crazy daughter' (Lazarre 1996, p. 28). Despite this familial acceptance, the racially nuanced maternal experience Lazarre (1976, 1996) captures in her two memoirs is poignant and painful.

Aspects of my life are both different and similar to those of Jordan, Lazarre and Jones. My parents were born in 1929 to recent-immigrant families. Although my mother's family struggled financially in Toronto, their attitudes reflected their petit bourgeois past in a small Polish city. My father's family origins are ambiguous; Canadian immigration records indicate that they were refugees escaping Russia through Romania in the early 1920s. Conflicting family stories and lack of birth documents leave us unsure. Growing up, I was inundated with stories of my maternal grandmother's sisters dying in Nazi extermination camps, my paternal great grandfather being killed in a pogrom, my dad being beat up by Quebecois kids, and how my stenographer mother could not get a job in Toronto's white Anglo-Saxon Protestant (WASP)-owned firms because Jews were restricted from participating in many areas of social life until the 1960s (Speisman 1979). Still, unlike some Jewish families who become very insular, my parents were sensitive to all forms of racism and had an admirable openness to others of different racial, cultural and class backgrounds. Although our extended families chose to live in Jewish neighbourhoods, my mother scorned the idea of living in 'middle-class Jewish ghettos'. Consequently, I grew up experiencing the subtle anti-Semitism of a predominantly middle-class genteel Anglo-Saxon midtown neighbourhood in the 1950s and 1960s. This unlikely environment for a Jewish child from a poor Yiddish-speaking, chaotic home fed my confusion, loneliness and discomfort with my Jewish identity. Compared to Jordan's experience with anti-Semitism in Virginia during the1930s,[9] my experience was far easier. Like Jones, who wanted a different life from her parents, I too hoped to find a place that felt like 'home'. With its strongly Jewish persona, I believed home could be found in New York City. After a year of planning, at twenty-two, elated by romanticism and rebelliousness, I crossed into the USA, travelling more kilometres than the actual distance between Toronto and New York.

As a teenager looking for an identity, I was fascinated with the music of Bessie Smith, Billie Holiday, Charles Mingus and John Coltrane, and the classic African-American writings of James Baldwin, Richard Wright and Ralph Ellison. As Lazarre (1996, p. xvi) writes, she 'discovered that African American literature often described [her] own deepest emotions, presenting a vision of the world and experience that was profoundly familiar to [her], a white, Jewish woman.' Her words could be my own. I believe other Jews, like Beat poet Allen Ginsberg (1956) who, in his poem, 'Howl', wrote of 'dragging themselves through [New York's] negro streets at dawn', relate to this as well. I read Leroi Jones, ignorant of the politics that had him change his name to Amiri Baraka and leave his Jewish wife. I pondered over the Martinique psychiatrist Frantz Fanon's (1967) discussion of anti-Semitism and anti-black racism, and became fascinated with the conflict between blacks and Jews that cultural and jazz critic Nat Hentoff (1970) of New York's *Village Voice* newspaper wrote of. I hoped that New York, the city whose Jewish and black cultural strands weaved together in my naive dreams, would create a new tapestry of my life. Moving to New York to explore the meaning of my Jewishness, love, marriage and children with an American black man shuttled me to a different exploration. This paper is the fruit of this dream.

Unlike my own experience, there is an implicit sense in Jordan, Lazarre and Jones's narratives that they feel 'other' from their interracial/inter-religious children. McBride (1996), a journalist, spent fourteen years trying to piece together his mother's otherness. As a child, he wondered where she came from and asked if she was white. She responded saying she was 'light skinned' and made by God. He recalls asking why she did not look like other mothers in their black neighbourhood:

> "Because I am not them," she says.
> "Who are you?" he asks.
> "I am your Mother."
> "Then why don't you look like Rodney's mother, or Pete's mother? How come you don't look like me?"
> "I do look like you, I am your mother." (McBride 1996, p. 12)

McBride noticed that his mother differed from other white people. She drank tea from a glass, conversed in Yiddish and did not trust 'outsiders' of either race. When, as an adult, he discovered her Jewish history, her differences became illuminated. He recalls: 'She never spoke of Jewish people as white people...she spoke about them as Jews' (McBride 1996, p. 87). Although they grew up in poor black neighbourhoods during the pre-bussing era[10], she insisted on sending them to predominantly white schools where they could receive a better education. Asking her if he was black or white, she snapped: 'You're a human being...educate yourself or you will be nobody!' When inquiring, 'Will I be a black nobody or just a nobody?', she answered dryly: 'If you are a nobody, it doesn't matter what colour you are.' To McBride (1996, p. 92), his mother's emphasis on education exemplified her Jewishness. Through Jordan's self-identified black Baptist son's narrative, we do not know if she too felt the 'racial otherness' we see with Lazarre and Jones.

Lazarre's children were raised with both knowledge and connection to their secular Jewish roots. Unlike Jordan, Lazarre grew up in New York, a safe social environment to be Jewish. Whether this contributed to her self-definition as white and why she and her husband initially defined the family as biracial, is difficult to conclude. Later, seeing their sons as phenotypically black, they decided that a biracial identity was not congruent with how their sons would be viewed. Poignantly, Lazarre (1996, p. 10) wonders if her sons ever regret having a white mother and if there is an 'unbridgeable distance' between them. She worries that her sons think of her as 'white' before they think of her as their 'Jewish mother, a natural fact of their identities.' She recalls her son telling her: 'I am black . . . I have a Jewish mother, but I am not bi-racial . . . a tragic mulatto.' Her attempt to say she understands is rebuffed with this painful response: 'I don't think you do, Mom. You can't understand this completely because you are white' (Lazarre 1996, p. 25). Turning inward, Lazarre (1996, p. 25) asks herself:

> What is this whiteness that threatens to separate me from my own child? Why haven't I seen it lurking, hunkering down, encircling me in some irresistible fog? I want to say the thing that will be most helpful to him, offer some carefully designed, unspontaneous permission for him to discover his own road, even if that means leaving me behind. On the other hand, I want to cry out, don't leave me, as he cried to me when I walked out of day-care centers, from baby-sitters, out of his first classroom in public school. And always, this double truth, as irresolvable as in any other passion, the paradox: she is me/not me; he is mine/not mine.

While the focus of Jones's (1990, p. 62) narrative is her marriage, like Lazarre, she too writes movingly about being the white Jewish mother of two interracial children. Acutely aware of her parents' disapproval, she feels guilty of 'the sin of breaking off the yoke' found in the *machzor*, the prayer book used during the Jewish High Holy Days. Although Jones's mother's rabbi grants permission for her to keep in touch with her transgressive daughter, she does so infrequently. For Jones, rejected by her family, and increasingly alienated by her husband's frequent reminders that 'one-half black makes you whole', Jones (1990, p. 52) ponders raising children: 'Could a white mother raise them? And white I would be, because I knew the Jews – mine at least – would give me up.' Still, Jones had the support of her in-laws who not only accepted and welcomed her, they also recognized her Jewish experience. Jesting, her mother-in-law would ask: 'Why this . . . wasn't being Jewish bad enough?' (Jones 1990, p. 108). We get a sense of this 'bad enough' when Jones (1990, p. 106) tells of her weekly experience on the way to visit her mother-in-law:

> There on the train, pair by pair, the eyes of the world drifted in and settled on us. Nothing can ready you for this . . . It felt, sitting there,

as if we were wearing a skin of public opinion, that stuck and clung and pressed and forced a change in the way you could breathe.

I feel that raising my children in Canada in the 1980s and 1990s mitigated the number of times I had to endure experiences like Jones describes above. Today, one commonly sees interracial couples and families in urban centres like Toronto or New York. Deborah and Valerie, the Jewish-Canadian mothers I interviewed,[11] feel that interracial unions are more accepted. Still, they share their racialized maternal experiences and tell me how religious differences add another layer of complexity. Although they are from a more tolerant generation, the issues they raise are remarkably similar to those in the narratives of Jordan, Jones, Lazarre and myself.

Deborah, a thirty-seven-year-old yoga teacher and writer, describes growing up in a down-to-earth, upper-middle-class, family-centred home in a 'pretty white and pretty Jewish' neighbourhood. Her father, a doctor, is the son of Polish-Jewish immigrants; her mother, a teacher then a stay-at-home mother, is the daughter of second-generation Russian Jews. Remembering back to elementary school, Deborah recalls only two black and three or four Asian classmates, plus her family's string of housekeepers, as the only people from racialized groups with whom she interacted. She says that race or racism was never discussed in her family; the one memory she has is of being upset by harsh reprimands from the family's black housekeeper. On telling her mother, Deborah is told to 'sympathize' because the housekeeper is going through a difficult time. In retrospect, Deborah wishes her mother had explained their housekeeper's life with more detail, perhaps explaining issues of social class and privilege. Saying little about the values she was raised with, she does say that she was she was always 'attracted to difficulty and cultural difference' during her high school years. When I ask why, she reflects:

> I feel like that's where I was always headed in a way, sometimes I imagine I was with someone who grew up like me and who was Jewish, and I sort of think I consciously shelved it, because even a lot of the guys I knew growing up, who might have been Jewish, they didn't have a similar experience to me, they were just different, right? Sometimes I just think about it . . . not like a rebellion, but just more conscious, and then there's the whole attraction thing, that's another element that you can't really plan for or predict.

Deborah does not discuss why she was attracted to her husband; she does discuss his 'cultural differences'. At age eleven, he, his three siblings and their mother immigrated to Canada from Jamaica and, although his parents were still married, his father stayed behind.

Deborah tells me of his harsh upbringing: first in Jamaica, then living in subsidized housing in downtown Toronto. After high school he attended a fashion programme that landed him a position in upscale menswear. Currently, he and Deborah live in downtown Toronto's arts community with their three-year-old son.

Valerie's life bears some similarity to Deborah's. Although ten years younger and single, she too is the mother of a three-year-old son. Valerie describes her mother as a first-generation Canadian, the daughter of Polish Holocaust survivors who immigrated to Canada shortly after the Second World War. She claims that because her maternal grandparents became financially successful, her mother never 'had to work' in either of the two careers – art teacher and architect – that she had trained for. Her father's family are third-generation Canadians with roots in Lithuania and Russia. After her parents' divorce when Valerie was in grade five, she lived between her father's home in a mixed suburb of Chinese, Jewish and 'just white people', and her mother's home in a mostly Jewish Toronto neighbourhood (where Deborah grew up). Although Valerie's family was not religiously observant, she attended Jewish primary day school. After grade six, she moved to a culturally and religiously diverse junior school followed by high school at one of Toronto's prestigious, international and inter-religious private girls' schools.

Valerie, like Deborah, says that as a child she had little exposure to people of other cultures and races. She remembers one friend of Asian descent whom she and her friends considered an 'honorary Jew'. Aside from this, she tells me that most families, including hers, had a Filipina nanny, which felt 'normal' and 'just the way things were for every-body'. While she does not recall race being discussed by her parents, she does remember them expressing sympathy towards victims of global issues such as genocide and war. Conversations with her grandparents were different:

> ...I remember as young as twelve or thirteen, I think once we all turned thirteen my bubbie and zaydie sat us down one at a time and gave us a talk about only dating Jewish people...they said it would be okay to be friends but you shouldn't get too close.

Thinking back, Valerie says that she did not interpret her grand-parents' conversation as racist or critical of other cultures; she saw it as 'just a normal Jewish thing' because so many Jews had lost their families in the Holocaust. Although she heard the occasional racist comment in her family, the extent of their racism was revealed when she became involved with her son's father. On receiving news of her pregnancy, her family vehemently opposed her having an interracial child. Suddenly, Valerie lost the emotional safety net of her close, loving, supportive family.

The theme of feeling emotionally unsafe or alone arises in the narratives of the mothers in my study to varying degrees. Without understating the frequency of family violence, most of us envision family life as a safe place where the challenges or vulnerabilities experienced in the social world are buffered by shared understanding and support. For Jewish mothers in interaccial or inter-religious families, shared understanding is often called into question, leaving these mothers feeling rejected, unsupported, alone or misunderstood by their families of origin, their children or their black partners. The theme of feeling competent as a mother is one place where this comes into play.

Valerie's experiences as a single mother exemplify the feelings I note above. She says she 'views parenting in a loving nurturing way' and that she 'just always thought of you know, raising this mixed kid, I just wanted him to feel really secure at home and safe and you know, in a loving environment.' She acknowledges that she sometimes feels unclear about what is best, and turns to her biracial friend for advice. In one heated argument, Valerie's friend tells her she is too 'nice' and 'easy-going' with her son. Admonishing, she racializes and stereotypes Valerie's maternal skills:

> He's going to think that he's entitled or he's going to go out there and act like any other [rich] Jewish kid but the world, but society is going to tell him otherwise and he's going to get a real smack in the face if you don't prepare him for it now.

Valerie says her friend's statement 'felt really uncomfortable', like she was being told she 'needs to change things about herself in order to raise him right.' Now she wonders if her mothering skills are 'wrong...like there is a whole different formula for a mixed kid' and worries that she will send her son out 'ill-prepared' to deal with issues of race that he may encounter. With no one to counterbalance her friend's opinion, Valerie feels insecure about her ability to be a good mother. Similar conflicts about raising a biracial son occur for Deborah as well.

I sense that Deborah feels uncomfortable telling me that issues of race arise when she and her husband discuss disciplining their son. Searching for the right words, she says:

> I feel like certain arguments that we might have had about parenting come down to race...but I learn something from it. I get his perspective, you know? But that's the only sort of issue that we've

had that has come down to race. Not come down to race, that's probably not the best way of saying it.

As if she is betraying a confidence, Deborah hesitantly tells me that her husband believes in 'harsh discipline', because their son is a black child who is going to be a black man in the world. Although her tone is unconvincing, she tells me that she understands 'what he's doing and why he's doing it and why he thinks it's important.' She says this 'satisfied the disagreement', enabling her to put aside her feeling that her husband was transferring his own harsh childhood treatment onto their son.

> It's just . . . I just felt that it was a point of understanding for me, like you as a black man are giving your child, who's also black, you know, mixed race, but black as well, your child, you're sort of like trying to shape him in a way for some of the tools you think he's going to need. Like it turned out to kind of be a positive thing for me, like a point of understanding, a point of him being responsible . . . just being realistic.

Deborah contrasts her parenting style and describes herself as nurturing. She feels her son benefits from this because he is a 'very warm child'. She thinks this has impacted on her husband's behaviour because she sees him 'softening'. Still, I sense Deborah is perturbed by their differences. She admits their 'conflict' gets 'heated' in moments and feels that this 'comes down to him being black'. Deborah adds that 'some biracial' people she knows with white mothers and black fathers seem to share her husband's beliefs. 'The mistake they feel the mum made,' she states, 'because it's always the mum's fault, is that yeah she just loved the kid, and just yeah didn't arm them . . . with the knowledge that they were black. I think that's usually the critique.' There is sarcasm in what she says that reveals an underlying hurt. Although she says her own and her husband's families support her mothering skills, I sense that, like the mothers in the narratives, she questions her maternal competence.

The narratives of Jordan, Lazarre, Jones, Valerie and Deborah begin to touch on the meaning and experiences of race for white Jewish birth mothers of children from interracial/inter-religious relationships. As Zack (1995) asserts, because racial cultures are learned and taught over generations, most people believe that race and racialized descriptions are factual and value-neutral categories. For the women in my research, the pressure of mothering across learned racial cultures creates conditions that can undermine or undervalue their maternal knowledge.

Conclusion

According to American psychologist and scholar of multiracial experience, Maria P.P. Root (2001), the birth of interracial children introduces issues that are usually irrelevant in mono-racial families. Concurring with Root, I add that additional issues arise when the family is also inter-religious. In my research, assumptions about white mothers of children from black/white interracial unions reflected in the literature were also reflected in the experiences of the white Jewish mothers in my study. Of these, three stand out: white mothers are 'other' to their interracial children; white mothers do not experience racism therefore can never understand or truly empathize with their interracial child's painful experiences of racism; and, white mothers are ill-equipped to socialize their black/white interracial children to withstand systemic racism.

For white/Jewish mothers, further issues are introduced. Miller and Miller's (1990) article on bridging the gap between African-American and white parenting styles of mothers of biracial children exemplifies this point. According to Miller and Miller (1990, p. 176) the availability of 'ethnically self-assertive [black] role models' and an 'ability to cope with the world from a [black] minority perspective' are crucial for the biracial child's developmental and mental health.[12] Given Jewish matrilineage, emphasis on black/white interracial children's paternal identity puts Jewish mothers in particular at odds with their own culture. Further, the implication that white mothers are unable to raise mentally healthy biracial children seems derisive. For phenotypically white Jewish mothers who may have had, or are likely to have, experiences of anti-Semitism either personaly or vicariously through relatives who survived or perished in the Holocaust, this feels particularly problematic. While Jewish mothers cannot share their children's experience of anti-black racism, to say that they do not experience the world from a 'minority perspective' whitewashes experiences of anti-Semitism.

Another assumption implicit in the literature is that black/white interracial relationships are mono-religious. Given the Christian hegemony of western countries, the majority of partners of Jewish women in interracial unions are Christian. For a Jewish mother, matrilineal hertiage and religious and cultural differences related to child-rearing may be as salient an issue as race is to her child's father. Just as she can be racialized as white, she can be constructed as 'religiously other' if conflicts arise with her child's father or his family. Also, in a union where the need for the children to identify as black dominates, the importance of a Jewish mother's own cultural identity may get overlooked, leaving her to feel both marginalized from her children and 'other' in her own home. These complex realities in the lives of Jewish mothers of black/white interracial children underscore the need for expanded ways of understanding and approaching women's life in families. As Bing and Trotman Reid (1996) assert, the portrayal of women and 'people of colour' in feminist psychological research often essentializes women's experiences and overlooks other socially constructed markers such as race, class, sexual orientation and gender, which also determine social placement and relative power. Bing and Trotman Reid (1991, p. 176) argue that because of the large numbers of 'unknown women' and 'unknowing research', 'further strategies are needed to begin to explain the needs and to hear the voices of the women who are still unknown in psychological research' (Bing and Trotman Reid, p. 192). For Jewish women in interracial/inter-religious relationships, I believe this is the case.

In closing, as a mother who once searched the literature for guidance, the opportunity to represent the voices of other mothers who have struggled with mothering across racialized boundaries is a privilege. Using life history and arts-informed research has allowed me to draw data from literary narrative, interviews and personal history to begin to tell the stories of a demographic group of women whose stories are rarely told. As Sameshima and Knowles (2008, p. 109) state:

> While the...research is informed by the arts it must ultimately address intellectual or other issues which make a contribution to a particular knowledge base...further, what is said...must be communicated in such a way that it offers possibilities for making a difference in peoples lives.

To this end, I hope my research on the experiences of race in the lives of Jewish-Canadian and Jewish-American birth mothers of children from black/white interracial inter-religious relationships makes a valuable contribution to our understanding of racialized motherhood.

Notes

1. My doctoral research at the Ontario Institute for Studies in Education, University of Toronto.
2. The term 'racialized' is relatively new. According to Tizard and Phoenix (2002, p. 6), this term clarifies the concept of 'race' as a socially constructed category rather than a biological reality. In this sense, 'racial meanings' are neither naturally occurring nor static, but rather, are dynamic social processes. My use of this term concurs with this view.
3. In the USA, where most current research on these families originates, the abolition of anti-miscegenation laws in 1967, the civil rights movement, affirmative action, and the inclusion of biracial and mixed-race categories in the US Census Bureau's racial classification system in 2000 (Root 2001) suggest continued growth and possible acceptance of this population. In Britain, Tizard and Phoenix's (2002) research found that attitudes

toward interracial unions have become more sympathetic. Canadian data found in the 2006 census (*Toronto Globe and Mail* 2008) and Canada's increased population from non-white countries (for a discussion of this, see AECMMT 1995) reflect a similar trend.

4.   For a comprehensive introduction to the troubled relationship between these two groups in the USA, see acclaimed Jewish-American jazz critic Nat Hentoff's (1970) edited book *Black Anti-Semitism and Jewish Racism*.

5.   Born of his curiosity about his mother's Jewish identity and early life as a Jewish woman in the South, James McBride's (1996) memoir draws on conversations with and research about her.

6.   Hettie Jones, author and teacher at the Graduate Writing Program of The New School in New York City, is a former chair of the PEN Prison Writing Committee, and the editor of *Aliens at the Border*, a collection of poetry her workshop at the Bedford Hills Correctional Facility.

7.   Leroi Jones (now known as Amiri Baraka) is a noted American writer of poetry, drama, fiction, essays and music criticism. He has frequently been criticized for his early writings, which were often misogynistic, homophobic, anti-white and anti-Semitic.

8.   Jane Lazarre is a writer and instructor at the New School for Social Research in New York. In 2003, she was a featured writer in the PBS documentary 'Matters of Race', produced and directed by Orlando Bagwell. Her writing has been the subject of critical works by many scholars including Susan Gubar, Jessica Benjamin, Maureen T. Reddy, Sara Ruddick, Joanne Frye and others.

9.   Jordan was called 'Jew baby' and 'Christ killer' (McBride 1996, p. 40).

10.   Busing refers to the desegregating practice of assigning and transporting students to schools in order to overcome the detrimental effects of racial and residential segregation on black children's' education.

11.   Deborah and Valerie are pseudonyms chosen to protect the identity of these participants.

12.   Miller and Miller (1990) cite studies on socialization and the black family.

References

AECMMT (ACCESS AND EQUITY CENTRE OF THE MUNICIPALITY OF METROPOLITAN TORONTO) 1995 *The Composition and Implications of Metropolitan Toronto's Ethnic, Racial and Linguistic Populations, 1991*, Toronto: Metropolitan Toronto Chief Administrator's Office

BARN, RAVINDER 1999 'White mothers, mixed-parentage children, and child welfare', *British Journal of Social Work*, vol. 29, no. 2, pp. 269–84

BING VANESSA M. and TROTMAN REID, PAMELA 1996 "Unknown women and unknowing research: consequences of colour and class in feminist psychology", in Nancy Goldberger *et al.* (eds), *Knowledge, Difference and Power: Essays Inspired by Women's Ways of Knowing*, New York: Basic Books, pp. 175–202

BRODKIN, KAREN 1998 *How Jews Became White Folks & What That Says about Race in America*, New Brunswick, NJ: Rutgers

CAUGHEY, JAMES L. 2006 *Negotiating Cultures and Identities: Life History Issues, Methods, and Readings*, Lincoln, NB: University of Nebraska Press

COLE, ARDRA L. and KNOWLES, J. GARY 2001 *Lives in Context: The Art of Life History Research*, Lanham, MD: Altamira Press

——— 2008 'Arts-informed research', in J. Gary Knowles and Ardra L. Cole (eds), *Handbook of the Arts in Qualitative Research*, Los Angelas: SAGE, pp. 55–81

COLLINS, PATRICIA HILL 1994 'Shifting the center: race, class, and feminist theorizing about motherhood', in Donna Bassin, Margaret Honey and Meryle M. Kaplan (eds), *Representations of Motherhood*, New Haven: Yale University, pp. 56–74

DELLAPERGOLA, SERGIO 2009 'Jewish out-marriage: a global perspective', in Shulamit Reinharz and Sergio DellaPergola (eds), *Jewish Intermarriage around the World*, New Brunswick, NJ: Transaction Publishers, pp. 13–39

EDWARDS, ROSALIND, *et al.* 2012 'Introduction: approaches to racial and ethnic mixedness and mixing', in Rosalind Edwards, *et al.* (eds), *International Perspectives on Racial and Ethnic Mixedness and Mixing*, Abingdon: Routledge, pp. 1–9

FANON, FRANTZ 1967 *Black Skin White Masks*, New York: Grove Press

FRANKENBERG, RUTH 1993 *White Women, Race Matters: The Social Construction of Whiteness*, Minneapolis, MN: University of Minnesota Press

GIBEL AZOULAY, KATYA 1997 *Black, Jewish and Interracial: It's Not the Color of Your Skin, But the Race of Your Kin, and Other Myths of Identity*, Durham, NC: Duke University Press

GINSBERG, ALLEN 1956 *Howl*, San Francisco: City Lights Books

GOLDSTEIN, BEVERLEY PREVATT 1999 'Black, with a white parent, a positive and achievable identity', *British Journal of Social Work*, vol. 29, no. 2, pp. 285–301

GREENE, BEVERLEY A. 1990 'What has gone before: the legacy of racism and sexism in the lives of black mothers and daughters', in Laura S. Brown and Maria P.P. Root (eds), *Diversity and Complexity in Feminist Therapy*, London: Harrington Park Press, pp. 207–23

HARMAN, VICKI 2010 'Experiences of racism and the changing nature of white privilege among lone white mothers of mixed-parentage children', *Ethnic and Racial Studies*, vol. 33, no. 2, pp. 176–94

HENTOFF, NAT 1970 *Black Anti-Semitism and Jewish Racism*, New York: Schocken

HILL, LAWRENCE 2001 *Black Berry, Sweet Juice: On Being Black and White in Canada*, Toronto: Harper Flamingo

HILL, MIRIAM R. and THOMAS, VOLKER 2000 'Strategies for racial identity development: narratives of black and white women in interracial partner relationships', *Family Relations*, vol. 49, no. 2, pp. 193–200

INFANTRY, ASHANTE 2000 'Multiracial balancing act: this is what Canadian looks like', *The Toronto Star*, 11 March, K1

JONES, HETTIE 1990 *How I Became Hettie Jones*, New York: Grove Press

LAZARRE, JANE 1976 *The mother knot*, Boston: Beacon Press

—— 1996 *Beyond the Whiteness of Whiteness: Memoir of a White Mother of Black Sons*, Durham, NC: Duke University Press

LUKE, CARMEN and LUKE, ALLAN 1999 'Theorizing interracial families and hybrid identity: an Australian perspective', *Educational Theory*, vol. 49, no. 2, pp. 223–49

MCBRIDE, JAMES 1996 *The Colour of Water: A Black Man's Tribute to his White Mother*, New York: Riverhead

MCKENZIE, LISA LOUISE 2009 'Finding value on a council estate: complex lives, motherhood, and exclusion', [PhD thesis, University of Nottingham. Available from: http://etheses.nottingham.ac.uk/1862/ [Accessed 6 December 2012]

MILLER, ROBIN G. and MILLER, BARBARA M. 1990 'Mothering the biracial child: bridging the gap between African American and white parenting styles', *Women and Therapy*, vol. 10, nos. 1–2, pp. 169–79

ROOT, MARIA P.P. (ed.) 1996 *The Multiracial Experience: Racial Borders as the New Frontier*, Thousand Oaks, CA: SAGE

—— 2001 *Love's Revolution: Interracial Marriage*, Philadelphia, PA: Temple University Press

SAMESHIMA, PAULINE and KNOWLES, J. GARY 2008 'Into artfulness: being grounded but not unbounded', in J. Gary Knowles, Sara Promislow and Ardra L. Cole (eds), *Creating Scholarartistry: Imagining the Arts-Informed Thesis or Dissertaion*, Halifax: Backalog Books, pp. 107–20

SENNA, DANZY 2004 'The mulatto millennium', in Jayne O. Ifekwunigwe (ed.), *'Mixed Race' Studies: A Reader*, London: Routledge, pp. 206–8

SPEISMAN, STEPHEN A. 1979 *The Jews of Toronto*, Toronto: McClelland and Stewart

SPICKARD, PAUL. R. 1989 *Mixed Blood: Intermarriage and Ethnic Identity in Twentieth-Century America*, Madison, WI: University of Wisconsin Press

TIZARD, BARBARA and PHOENIX, ANN 2002 *Black, White or Mixed Race? Race and Racism in the Lives of Young People of Mixed Heritage*, London: Routledge

INFANTRY, A. 2000 'Multiracial balancing act: This is what Canadian looks like', *The Toronto Star*, 3 April, k1

VERBIAN, CHANNA 2006 'White birth mothers of black/white biracial children: addressing racialized discourses in feminist and multicultural literature', *Journal of the Association for Research on Mothering*, vol. 8, no. 1&2, pp. 213–22

WEEKS, C. 2008 'Interracial relationships rise 30% in five years', *The Toronto Globe and Mail*, 3 April, L1

WINDDANCE TWINE, FRANCE 2004 'A white side of black Britain: the concept of racial literacy', *Ethnic and Racial Studies*, vol. 27, no. 6, pp. 878–907

WINKS, ROBIN W. 1997 *The Blacks in Canada*, 2nd edn, Montreal: McGill-Queens University Press

ZACK, NAOMI 1995 'Introduction', in Naomi Zack (ed.), *American Mixed Race: The Culture of Microdiversity*, London: Rowan and Littlefield, pp. xv–xxv

Researching white mothers of mixed-parentage children: the significance of investigating whiteness

Joanne Britton

Abstract

This article takes as its starting point the increasing number of research studies that pay specific attention to family relationships when investigating mixedness. It draws on the critical study of whiteness to illustrate the significance of examining, in more detail than is usual, white mothers' racialized identity in studies of mixed-parentage families. It is argued that by doing so, understanding of the identity development and sense of belonging of children and young people in mixed-parentage families can be enhanced, as well as understanding of these issues in mixed-parentage families generally. The article explains how kinship relationships and wider social networks are two related areas of investigation that can help to shed light on what happens to whiteness in mixed-parentage families. Both encourage a specific focus on the identity and sense of belonging of mothers, without marginalizing the identities of other family members.

The development of 'mixed race' studies in recent years has ensured that the issue of mixedness is now firmly on the research agenda for social scientists investigating race and racism (Parker and Song 2001). In the British context, studies of mixed race have paid most attention to mixed-parentage children and adults with one white parent and one parent of African/Caribbean origin (e.g. Ifekwunigwe 1999; Christian 2000; Tizard and Phoenix 2001; Twine 2004). This is partly due to their relatively large number in the mixed-parentage population, yet also reflects the centrality of the binary division of black and white to the historical development of racism, and the resulting development of dominant, common-sense notions of mixedness. A key focus of research has been the identity development of children and young people of mixed parentage (Ifekwunigwe 1999; Tizard and Phoenix 2001; Olumide 2002; Ali 2003; Barn and Harman 2006). The significance of the identity of white mothers of mixed-parentage children has not tended to be a focus of investigation, with the resulting inference that it is of little relevance in understanding issues of belonging and identity in mixed-parentage families.

There are, however, an increasing number of research studies that pay specific attention to family relationships (Twine 1999, 2000, 2004; Tyler 2005; Cabellero, Edwards and Puthussery 2008; Song 2010). This broadened focus has included exploring the experiences of white mothers of mixed-parentage children and studies have investigated how they manage what Jill Olumide (2002, p. 4) refers to as their family's 'mixed race condition' (Twine 1999, 2000, 2004; Harman 2010; McKenzie 2010). They have has also drawn attention to the importance of considering the interaction between race, ethnicity, gender, social class and place in seeking to understand the mothers' experiences. In doing so, a key contribution of these studies has been to begin to highlight the relevance of whiteness to the mothers' experiences and family relationships.

This article draws on the critical study of whiteness to illustrate the significance of investigating further white mothers' racialized identity in studies of mixed-parentage families. It is argued that investigating whiteness in this way will enhance understanding of the identity development and sense of belonging of children and young people in mixed-parentage families, as well as understanding of these issues in mixed-parentage families generally. Whiteness is conceived of here as a marked racialized identity that only exists in relation to other racialized identities, such as blackness (Garner 2007, p. 2). However, as Byrne (2006, p. 3) explains 'whiteness is more than a conscious identity, it is also a position within racialised discourses as well as a set of practices and imaginaries.' As such, it is also relevant to the ethnic, classed and gendered identities expressed by white mothers of mixed-parentage children. Lastly, whiteness 'is a location of structural advantage in societies structured by racial dominance' (Frankenberg 1993, p. 1). Three key overarching questions arise from this conception of whiteness, all of which require further empirical investigation in order to build on the findings of previous studies. How does the white racialized identity of white mothers of mixed-parentage children exist in relation to the racialized identities of their children and other family members? What part does whiteness play in the racialized, ethnic, classed and gendered identities that they express and how is it practised and imagined in relation to parenting? To what extent and in what circumstances do they relinquish or retain the so-called 'invisible knapsack' of white privilege for themselves and their children

(McKintosh 1998)? Addressing these questions can enhance under-standing of what happens to whiteness in mixed-parentage families, both in terms of the identity and sense of belonging of family members and the playing out of racialized relationships of power within the family and beyond.

This article explains how kinship relationships and wider social networks are two related areas of investigation that can help to address these questions. It is argued that they are particularly fruitful because they allow investigation of white mothers' racialized identity without marginalizing the identities of other family members. The mothers' relationships with significant others, including, for example, their partner and/or father of their children, become an important focus. Before exploring kinship relationships and social networks, the article critically discusses dominant notions of the good mother and provides an explanation of the relevance of the critical study of whiteness, as a basis for exploring the racialized identity of white mothers of mixed-parentage children.

Whiteness and the good mother

In considering the significance of their racialized identity, it is useful to reflect on how white mothers of mixed-parentage children are positioned in relation to dominant social and cultural understandings of good mothering. It has been widely documented that, historically, white mothers of mixed-parentage children, and their relationships, have faced racialized social censoring and controls as a consequence of them straying from dominant racialized social norms (Benson 1981; Ware 1992; Katz 1996). Social norms are defined as codes to acceptable and moral behaviour and behaving in a morally acceptable way is regarded as key to belonging to a society or social group (Goffman 1959; May 2008, pp. 471–2). Although the extent and nature of social censoring and controls has changed over time, the behaviour of white mothers of mixed-parentage children is, arguably, morally doubtful because they are seen to have transgressed dominant social norms. It follows that the quality of their mothering can be called into question as a consequence.

Questions about the quality of their mothering are related to the socially and culturally situated nature of motherhood, meaning that what is defined as good or bad mothering is dependent upon the specific social and cultural context in which mothering takes place (Richardson 1993). All mothers negotiate their role through idealized standards that are culturally prescribed and, in doing so, their subjectivity is produced through the playing out of gendered, classed and racialized social norms (Byrne 2006, p. 117). This cultural idealization of motherhood helps to explain why white mothers of mixed-parentage children can be , Edwards and Puthusseryseen to betray prevailing social and cultural representations of the 'good mother'. The socially valued position of good mother is understood to be less available to women who are seen to have deviated from or transgressed dominant social norms. As May (2008, p. 473) has argued, these norms dictate that a good mother is, for example, heterosexual and is married to or cohabiting with the father of her children. The same norms can result in an understanding that a good mother chooses the man who will be the father of her children from the same, or at least a similar, ethnic and racialized background to herself. Research evidence indicates that white mothers of mixed-parentage children are confronted with a critical, racialized social gaze that does not fall upon white mothers in racially homogeneous families (Twine 2000; Cabellero, Edwards and Puthussery 2008; Harman 2010). Their parenting is scrutinized, found to be deficient and, as a result, they adopt various strategies to demonstrate their maternal competence (Twine 2000; Harman 2010). When seeking to present themselves as good mothers, white mothers of mixed-parentage children are therefore faced with a specific challenge that is not faced by white mothers in racially homogeneous relationships.

Despite this, it is important not to overstate the commonality of experience among white mothers of mixed-parentage children as the extent to which they are able to present themselves as good mothers is similarly influenced by a range of other factors, including social class background and whether or not they are single parents. In her study of white mothers of mixed-parentage children, Harman (2010, p. 188) found that 'mothers described being assumed to be single by strangers, presumed to be sexually available and seen as a threat by women that they might "steal" their partner.' These assumptions highlight the interplay of class, gender and race in the formation of stereotypical understandings about white mothers of mixed-parentage children and echo research that has shown how working-class women are rendered valueless, sexually promiscuous and potentially dangerous (Skeggs 1997; McKenzie 2010). White mothers of mixed-parentage children are subjected to a critical gaze that is therefore classed, gendered and racialized and the extent to which their mothering is regarded as deficient is dependent on the specific social and cultural context in which it occurs. However, regardless of their differences, it is clear that the social advantages of whiteness are not straightforwardly accrued for this group of white women.

The (in)visibility of whiteness

Whiteness is described as an empty category, socially and politically constructed as having no content and therefore unseen (e.g.

Frankenberg 1993; Dyer 1997). It is argued that much of the power of whiteness lies in its ability to escape definition while systematically defining the 'other' at the same time (Bonnett 2000). This means that whiteness is generally invisible to those categorized socially as white and, as a consequence, the advantages of whiteness remain unseen as well (Garner 2007, pp. 35–9). Following from this, it has been argued that white women are usually unaware of their whiteness and white privileges, and the part they play in protecting and perpetuating them, even though their thoughts and actions are structured by whiteness (Frankenberg 1993, p. 1–22). However, Frankenberg (1993), described 'moments of questioning' in which white women become aware of their whiteness and its consequences. Research has highlighted that racism is a new experience for white mothers of mixed-parentage children, who report incidences of abuse, harassment and discrimination directed at both themselves and their children (Banks 1996; Barn 1999; Harman 2010). White mothers of mixed-parentage children may, as a consequence of these specific experiences, have 'moments of questioning' in which their whiteness becomes apparent. This is suggested by the results of Harman's (2010, p. 188) study as 'many mothers felt that their experiences of racism were not fully recognized as they are white.'

It is also possible that their whiteness is made visible to both themselves and others in new and challenging ways at a more mundane, day-to-day level. A study of white women who are Muslim and choose to wear the *hijab* indicated how they became aware of, and indeed distanced from, the normative status and associated privileges of whiteness as a consequence of being 'otherized' through observing Islamic dress codes (Franks 2000, p. 927). Their experiences of everyday encounters with other white people included racist abuse, becoming the source of social embarrassment and avoidance, and being incorrectly identified as a non-English speaker (Franks 2000). Like these women, white mothers of mixed-parentage children are confronted with a critical, racialized social gaze that potentially disputes and undermines their claims to a privileged white identity. This raises questions about the extent to which white mothers of mixed-parentage children are able to retain the social privileges of whiteness, and also provides a reminder of the difficulties that they may face in presenting themselves socially as good mothers.

The dominant everyday view of racialized identities is that they have a permanent essence that is fixed and inevitably sets one racialized group apart from another (Miles and Brown 2003, p. 75). France Winddance Twine's (2000, 2010) research on white mothers of children of African descent illustrates this understanding as it reveals how they and their children are categorized and judged according to essentialist understandings. Twine's research examined the views that black family members expressed about the white mothers in their mixed-parentage families. She found that the mothers were perceived to be unable to empathize with their children and incapable of dealing effectively with the children's experiences of racism (Twine 2000, pp. 83–9). Not only this, unlike black mothers, the white mothers in these families were required to prove their maternal competence in parenting children categorized socially as black and this included their children being evaluated for black cultural competence on the basis of learned cultural behaviours (Twine 2000, p. 103). These findings alert us to the significance of considering how white family members view mothers of mixed-parentage children. Are the mothers similarly perceived as unable to empathize with their children and incapable of dealing effectively with the children's experiences of racism? Are they also evaluated according to if and how far their children display white cultural competence and learned cultural behaviours that are regarded as white? The latter is particularly important given the relevance of white cultural competence and behaviour as an important precondition for obtaining the privileges of whiteness.

This draws our attention to how the white racialized identity of white mothers of mixed-parentage children exists in relation to the racialized identities of their children and other family members. It raises questions about the extent to which whiteness, as a set of discourses, practices and imaginaries, is present in their parenting and about how they, intentionally and unintentionally, relinquish or retain the privileges of whiteness. It also highlights how both blackness and whiteness are implicated in the everyday negotiation of racialized identity and belonging, and reinforces that exploring whiteness is essential to understanding how white mothers of mixed-parentage children manage their family's racialized diversity. The following sections explore how kinship relationships and wider social networks provide a useful way of studying this empirically.

Kinship relationships

Kinship is highly relevant to investigating further issues of identity and belonging in mixed-parentage families as it remains one of the most important sources of enduring individual primary identity and is considered a principal bond between people that is most resistant to change (Jenkins 1996, p. 64). In everyday terms, kinship groups are seen as networks of social relationships that are bound together by well-defined customs, rights and obligations. A UK study on parenting 'mixed' children indicated the significance of kinship in mixed-parentage families. It found that nearly all of the parents who participated in the research cited family history and cultural traditions or way of life as the most important issues to pass on to their children to give them a sense of who they are (Caballero, Edwards and Puthussery 2008, pp. 15–16). Similarly, studies of mixed-parentage people and families have highlighted the significance of heritage, and the composite issues of descent, origins and genealogy, to their identity formation and sense of belonging (Tizard and Phoenix 2001; Ali 2003; Twine 2004; Tyler 2005). They have shed light on how people of mixed parentage and their parents make sense of biological and cultural relatedness in order to understand and accommodate their family's different racial origins and identities.

These studies have made a valuable contribution to understanding of identity and belonging in mixed-parentage families and have indicated the usefulness of considering the relevance of whiteness in making sense of biological and cultural relatedness. In doing so, it is useful to consider how the blurring of analytical boundaries between the biological and cultural in studies of kinship has led to this focus on 'relatedness' – drawing attention to the continuous process of how people become connected to others, particularly through everyday practices (Carsten 2000, pp. 2–18). Investigating 'relatedness' serves to raise questions about the part played by whiteness, as a set of discourses, practices and imaginaries, in the everyday processes and interactions that connect people in mixed-parentage families along kinship lines. With specific reference to white mothers of mixed-parentage children, this entails foregrounding the relevance of their racialized identity to how they manage their family's racialized diversity. Focusing on kinship relationships therefore provides a way of exploring how and in what circumstances whiteness comes into play when white mothers address the key parenting issues of identity and belonging.

It is important to stress that interrogating the significance of whiteness is most straightforwardly achieved through an investigation of white mothers' relationships with other family members who are regarded as significant kin. This reinforces how the white racialized identity of white mothers of mixed-parentage children exists in relation to the racialized identities of other family members. First and foremost, it entails focusing on the mother's relationship with her partner and/or father of her children and involves considering how they approach the challenge of incorporating children into kinship trajectories that are seemingly incompatible because they differ along ethnic and racial lines. In particular, it is essential to consider if, how and in what circumstances whiteness is privileged in the negotiation of kinship relationships between parents. This can help to address the claim that we still know relatively little about how parents from different ethnic and racial backgrounds negotiate their children's sense of identity and belonging (Caballero, Edwards and Puthussery 2008).

The mothers', and indeed fathers', relationship with grandparents and the contribution they make in developing kinship relationships in mixed-parentage families is also potentially significant. For white mothers of mixed-parentage children, relying on grandparents for practical and emotional support has been shown to be complicated by racism so grandparents' potential contribution should not be over-stated (Twine 1999; Harman 2010, p. 183). Although the contribution of grandparents cannot be presumed, particularly as this risks privileging biological connectedness in studying kinship relationships, studies have shown that adopted children spend more time with their grandparents than biological children and it has been argued that this is one deliberate way of incorporating children into their parents' kinship trajectories (Howell 2003, p. 475). It would be useful to investigate if this is also the case for children of mixed parentage and, in interrogating whiteness, it would be particularly useful to investigate if, how and when kinship relationships with white grandparents are privileged. In fact, it would be useful to investigate this in relation to any white kin identified as significant by mothers. This includes considering if and in what circumstances developing and privileging connections with white kin reflects white mothers' awareness of the social advantages of whiteness and if it represents a strategy for retaining these advantages and attempting to pass them on to the children. On the other hand, it is also useful to investigate the extent to which fostering relationships with kin who are not white is understood to contribute to relinquishing some of the privileges of whiteness.

Wider social networks

Social networks are commonly defined as sets of social relationships between people who understand themselves to share specific social ties; they usually involve friendship, advice and information exchange and practical and emotional support. Individuals and families rely on people in their wider social networks for these kinds of exchanges and support so it makes sense to investigate relationships that white mothers of mixed-parentage children develop with other people who they do not identify as kin but nevertheless regard as important to them and their family. In doing so, it is important to consider that hierarchy is deeply embedded in social practice and, as a result, people's social networks tend to lack diversity in terms of the social class, gender and ethnic and racial backgrounds of the people who make them up (Bottero and Irwin 2003, p. 473). As we tend to associate with people from similar ethnic and racial backgrounds to ourselves, whom we are friends with and whom we marry and have relationships with is therefore strongly influenced by our ethnic and racial background. It can be hypothesized that, in reflecting the family's diversity, the social networks of white mothers of mixed parentage are likely to be characterized by greater diversity than is usual. Empirical investigation is therefore valuable in shedding light on the composition, nature and consequences of the social networks to which they belong.

Specifically, the part that whiteness plays in connecting white mothers and their families to people socially becomes an important focus of investigation. This involves considering if, how and in what circumstances whiteness, as a set of discourses, practices and imaginaries, is relevant to their participation in particular social networks. It also includes examining if, how and in what circumstances whiteness is privileged in the fostering of these networks and if and the extent to which white mothers see this as a way of retaining the advantages of whiteness and securing them for their children. On the other hand, the potential for white mothers of mixed-parentage children to relinquish some of the privileges of whiteness as a result of marginalization or exclusion from particular social networks can also be investigated. Examining the diversity of social networks necessarily involves considering the relative significance of networks in which whiteness is not privileged as well. These include networks in which people share the ethnic or racial background of the father and those that include other white mothers of mixed-parentage families or mixed-parentage families generally. The significance that white mothers attribute to these different social networks can provide an important insight into what happens to whiteness in mixed-parentage families, in relation to the racialized identities of family members, parenting practices and experiences, and the operation of racialized privilege.

In terms of understanding the identity development and sense of belonging of people of mixed parentage, the influence of social networks and ties with people of each parent's heritage and other people of mixed race is arguably a key question for policy makers. This reinforces the usefulness of examining the various social networks in which white mothers of mixed-parentage children and their families are involved and, by implication, supports the argument that the relevance of whiteness should not be ignored.

Conclusion

The overall aim of this article has been to explain why the racialized identity of white mothers of mixed-parentage children is of key relevance to understanding issues of identity and belonging in mixed-parentage families. It has drawn attention to the significance of focusing on whiteness, as a position within racialized discourses, a set of practices and imaginaries and a location of structural advantage, to further illuminate our understanding of mixed-parentage families (Frankenberg 1993; Byrne 2006). It is perhaps unsurprising that whiteness has been marginalized in studies of mixed-parentage families, given that it is commonly described as an empty category that escapes definition and remains unseen (Frankenberg 1993; Dyer 1997). Whiteness is present in everyday social practices, processes and interactions, yet there is an assumption, sometimes implicit and at other times explicit, that it is unimportant to the identity development of mixed-parentage children. By uncovering what happens to whiteness in families in which one parent is categorized normatively as white, we are arguably in a better position to understand the meaning and role of race and racism in the lives of all members of mixed-parentage families.

A tighter focus on whiteness encourages the inclusion of white fathers of mixed-parentage children in future research. White fathers are a numerically less significant group in the British context and have been notably absent from the research agenda. It would be interesting to consider how successful they are in retaining the privileges of whiteness in comparison to white mothers. Likewise, the role of black fathers has been consistently neglected in studies of mixed-parentage families and this is likely to reflect the traditional, restricted focus on white single mothers. This article has explained how focusing on kinship and social networks enables investigation of the relevance of white mothers' racialized identity without excluding that of other family members. Examining the role of fathers generally and the related interplay of race and gender in shaping relationships between family members also helps to ensure that a commonality of experience in mixed-parentage families is not overstated.

Considering what happens to whiteness in families of mixed parentage in which one parent is categorized normatively as white has implications for our theoretical understanding of both mixed race and whiteness. This is important because there has been a tendency for these two specialisms within ethnic and racial studies to develop in parallel, without significant overlap. It is one way in which the critical study of whiteness and mixed race studies can inform and enlighten each other and, together, they can contribute further to our understanding of contemporary forms of racism. This includes interrogating the potential for taken-for-granted racial categories to be undermined and essentialist notions of racial difference to be challenged.

'Mixaphobia' has been defined as a contemporary distrust of mixing connected to the apparent failures of integration and associated critique of multiculturalism (Bauman 2003). This contemporary phenomenon sits uneasily alongside the growing mixed-parentage population so the greater social acceptance and, sometimes superficial, celebration of mixing does not automatically herald the demise of the hierarchical category of race. Likewise, so-called 'new wave' accounts of mixedness emphasize that people who are mixed are not 'mixed up', but rather perceive their identities as flexible and multiple, yet secure. Rather, their problems lie with how others view their mixedness (Caballero, Haynes and Tikly 2007, p. 346). All of this serves as a reminder that a better understanding of issues of identity and belonging in mixed-parentage families can help to challenge the persisting distrust of mixing. This article has explained why a tighter focus on whiteness should be a key part of this endeavour.

References

ALI, S. 2003 *Mixed-Race, Post-Race: Gender, New Ethnicities and Cultural Practices*, Oxford: Berg

BANKS, N. 1996 'Young single white mothers with black children in therapy', *Clinical Child Psychology and Psychiatry*, vol. 1, no. 1, pp. 19–28

BARN, R. 1999 'White mothers, mixed-parentage children and child welfare', *British Journal of Social Work*, vol. 29, no. 2, pp. 269–84

BARN, R. and HARMAN, V. 2006 'A contested identity: an exploration of the competing social and political discourse concerning the identification and positioning of young people of inter-racial parentage', *British Journal of Social Work*, vol. 36, no. 8, pp. 1309–24

BAUMAN, Z. 2003 *Liquid Love: On the Fragility of Human Bonds*, London: Polity Press

BENSON, S. 1981 *Ambiguous Ethnicity: Interracial Families in London*, New York: Cambridge University Press

BONNETT, A. 2000 *White Identities*, Harlow: Pearson

BOTTERO, W. and IRWIN, S. 2003 'Locating difference: class, "race" and gender, and the shaping of social inequalities', *Sociological Review*, vol. 51, no. 4, pp. 463–83

BYRNE, B. 2006 *White Lives: The Interplay of 'Race', Class and Gender in Everyday Life*, London: Routledge

CABALLERO, C., EDWARDS, R. and PUTHUSSERY, S. 2008 *Parenting 'Mixed' Children: Negotiating Differences and Belonging in Mixed Race, Ethnicity and Faith Families*, York: Joseph Rowntree Foundation

CABALLERO, C., HAYNES, J. and TIKLY, L. 2007 'Researching mixed race in education: perceptions, policies and practices', *Race, Ethnicity and Education*, vol. 10, no. 3, pp. 345–62

CARSTEN, J. 2000 'Introduction', in J. Carsten (ed.), *Cultures of Relatedness: New Approaches to the Study of Kinship*, Cambridge: Cambridge University Press, pp. 1–36

CHRISTIAN, M. 2000 *Multiracial Identity: An International Perspective*, Basingstoke: MacMillan Press

DYER, R. 1997 *White*, London: Routledge

FRANKENBERG, R. 1993 *White Women, Race Matters: The Social Construction of Whiteness*, London: Routledge

FRANKS, M. 2000 'Crossing the borders of whiteness? White Muslim women who wear the hijab in Britain today', *Ethnic and Racial Studies*, vol. 23, no. 5, pp. 917–29

GARNER, S. 2007 *Whiteness: An Introduction*, London: Routledge

GOFFMAN, E. 1959 *The Presentation of Self in Everyday Life*, New York: Anchor Books Doubleday

HARMAN, V. 2010 'Experiences of racism and the changing nature of white privilege among lone white mothers of mixed-parentage children in the UK', *Ethnic and Racial Studies*, vol. 33, no. 2, pp. 176–94

HOWELL, S. 2003 'Kinning: the creation of life trajectories in transnational adoptive families', *Journal of the Royal Anthropological Institute*, vol. 9, no. 3, pp. 465–84

IFEKWUNIGWE, J. O. 1999 *Scattered Belongings: Cultural Paradoxes of Race, Nation and Gender*, London: Routledge

JENKINS, R. 1996 *Social Identity*, London: Routledge

KATZ, I. 1996 *The Construction of Racial Identity in Children of Mixed Parentage: Mixed Metaphors*, London: Jessica Kingsley

MCINTOSH, P. 1988 *White Privilege and Male Privilege: A Personal Account of Coming to See Correspondences through Work in Women's Studies*, Working Paper 189, Wellesley, MA: Wellesley College

MCKENZIE, L. L. 2010 'Finding value on a council estate: complex lives, motherhood and exclusion', [PhD thesis, University of Nottingham. Available from: http://etheses.nottingham.ac.uk/1862/ [Accessed 6 December 2012]]

MAY, V. 2008 'On being a "good" mother: the moral presentation of self in written life stories', *Sociology*, vol. 42, no. 3, pp. 470–86

MILES, R. and BROWN, M. 2003 *Racism*, 2nd edn, London: Routledge

OLUMIDE, J. 2002 *Raiding the Gene Pool: The Social Construction of Mixed Race*, London: Pluto Press

PARKER, D. and SONG, M. (eds) 2001 *Rethinking 'Mixed Race'*, London: Pluto Press

RICHARDSON, D. 1993 *Women, Motherhood and Childrearing*, Basingstoke: MacMillan Press

SKEGGS, B. 1997 *Formations of Class and Gender*, London: SAGE

―――― 2010 'Is there "a" mixed race group in Britain? The diversity of multiracial identification and experience', *Critical Social Policy*, vol. 30, no. 3, pp. 337–58

TIZARD, B. and PHOENIX, A. 2001 *Black, White or Mixed Race? Race and Racism in the Lives of Young People of Mixed Parentage*, 2nd edn, London: Routledge

TWINE, F. W. 1999 'Bearing blackness in Britain: the meaning of racial difference for white mothers of African-descent children', *Social Identities: Journal of Race, Culture and Nation*, vol. 5, no. 2, pp. 185–210

―――― 2000 'Bearing blackness in Britain: the meaning of racial difference for white birth mothers of African-descent children', in H. Ragone and F. W. Twine (eds), *Ideologies and Technologies of Motherhood: Race, Class, Sexuality, Nationalism*, London: Routledge, pp. 76–110

―――― 2004 'A white side of black Britain: the concept of racial literacy', *Ethnic and Racial Studies*, vol. 27, no. 6, pp. 878–907

―――― 2010 *A White Side of Black Britain: Interracial Intimacy and Racial Literacy*, Durham, NC: Duke University Press

TYLER, K. 2005 'The genealogical imagination: the inheritance of interracial identities', *The Sociological Review*, vol. 5, no. 3, pp. 476–94

WARE, V. 1992 *Beyond the Pale: White Women, Racism and History*, London: Verso

Social capital and the informal support networks of lone white mothers of mixed-parentage children

Vicki Harman

Abstract

This paper draws upon in-depth interviews with thirty lone white mothers of mixed-parentage children in Britain in order to analyse the range of informal support networks that mothers utilize in their parenting. The findings show that while racism impacted upon mothers' support networks, their parenting experiences also led to an impetus to enlarge these networks, for example through support groups, friendships with people from minority ethnic backgrounds and other interracial families. The close friendships between lone white mothers of mixed-parentage children were particularly valued for non-judgemental support and empathy and it is argued that they constitute a form of bonding capital.

Introduction

This paper considers the parenting experiences of lone white mothers of mixed-parentage children and examines the perceptions that they have of their informal support networks. Key questions to be addressed are: what are the informal support networks utilized by lone white mothers of mixed-parentage children?; and how do race and ethnicity influence the support networks available to mothers? The inclusion of a 'mixed' group on the 2001 census led to the recognition of increasing numbers of children with parents from different ethnic backgrounds in Britain. Lucinda Platt's (2009) analysis of the Labour Force Survey data 2004–08 showed that around

85 per cent of people in Britain described themselves as white British and the mixed group accounted for 1.1 per cent of the population. While the mixed group accounts for a relatively small proportion of the population as a whole, it comprises a significant proportion of the minority ethnic population (Owen 2005). Black Caribbean men and women were particularly likely to be in an interracial relationship, with 48 per cent of partnered black Caribbean men and 34 per cent of partnered women in such a relationship (Platt 2009). Furthermore, the mixed group is a young population, with the majority of mixed-ethnicity children under sixteen (Platt 2009). Data from the Labour Force Survey suggests that 51 per cent of children who were categorized as mixed white and black Caribbean live in lone parent families (Platt 2009, p. 34). As a significant family type for this group of children, it is important that the circumstances in which lone mothers parent their children are understood.

Parenting and support networks

Within the literature on parenting, a considerable number of studies have demonstrated that the social networks available to families have important implications for their well-being and parents' ability to cope with parenting (Ghate and Hazel 2002; Gardner 2003; Attree 2005; Barn et al., 2006; Barnes 2007). Furthermore, the perception of being supported has been shown to be as important as the tangible support received (Attree 2005). Lone parents in general are recognized as facing a number of structural difficulties such as low income, poor housing and poor health, as well as social disapproval (Rowlingson and McKay 2002). A study of families parenting in 'poor environments' found that 60 per cent of lone parents said they would like more support, compared to thirty 39 per cent of parents with partners (Ghate and Hazel 2002). In many cases, lone parents appear to lose out on support that would have been provided from the father and his family. Instead, the lone mother's own mother was found to be an important source of support (Ghate and Hazel 2002). It has been suggested that lone white mothers of mixed-parentage children could be vulnerable to experiencing a lack of support. For example, inadequate support networks have been put forward as one possible explanatory factor for the over-representation of children from this family background in the public care system (Barn 1999). Social capital provides a theoretical tool to help shed light on the formation and maintenance of friendship and family relationships. This concept will now be introduced in more detail.

Social capital

According to Robert Putnam (1995, p. 67), social capital refers to the 'features of social organization such as networks, norms, and social trust that facilitate coordination and cooperation for mutual benefit.' This means that the networks that people have – their connections to other people – are valuable. The notion that social capital is declining in modern American and British society has dominated much of the social capital literature (Halpern 2005). In terms of social policy, social capital became a popular concept under the New Labour administration in the UK, underpinning discourses concerning regeneration (Edwards, Franklin and Holland 2003). It can also be argued to be a relevant concept at the current time given David Cameron's emphasis on the 'big society' and the assumption that members of the public will be increasingly active in their local communities as public services are cut back. Within the social capital literature there are competing views on whether families are central to the formation of social capital or are merely implicated in the process (Edwards, Franklin and Holland 2003).

Social capital has been identified as having bonding, bridging and linking functions (Halpern 2005). 'Bonding' refers to networks and relationships that reinforce trust and values within a group. Bonding ties are made with people who are similar to oneself. 'Bridging' social capital is outward looking, referring to contact, trust and reciprocity between members of different groups. Finally, 'linking' social capital refers to relationships that allow individuals to link across formal and informal resources. Later in this paper I consider the particular manifestations of these functions for lone white mothers of mixed-parentage children. For Bourdieu (1987), social capital is comprised of social obligations that can, under some circumstances, be converted to economic capital. Social capital is thus a form of investment in the community, which is likely to provide some benefit for participants at a later date (Bourdieu 1987). While Bourdieu's work recognizes that social capital can operate to maintain the status quo, the work of the classic proponents of social capital, such as Coleman and Putnam, has been criticized for not paying sufficient attention to the role of ethnicity and other key social divisions in shaping social networks (Reynolds 2010). However, in his more recent work Robert Putnam (2007) has explored the influence of ethnic diversity and immigration on social capital with some worrying conclusions. His analysis of US survey data suggests that inhabitants of diverse communities tend to withdraw from social life and to have less faith in their local community and its leaders, concluding that 'Diversity, at least in the short run, seems to bring out the turtle in all of us' (Putnam 2007, pp. 150–1). More evidence is needed to test the parameters of these findings and to understand the processes underpinning the outcomes that Putnam describes. While this paper cannot offer macro-level conclusions about the effects of ethnicity and social capital, it will offer valuable qualitative insights into the experiences of a group for whom ethnic diversity is often an integral part of everyday life.

Interracial families in Britain and their support networks

In general, support networks have not been a major focus of the research on interracial families. While topics such as identity have received more attention, some studies conducted over the last thirty years have elicited important information about the wider kinship and friendship networks in which families are embedded and these studies will now be introduced. Wilson (1981, 1987) studied the identity of fifty-one mixed-parentage children (aged six to nine years old) living with their parents. She pointed to mothers' experiences of marginality due to the experience of racism and the lack of acceptance from others (Wilson 1981). She found that the white mothers who were most successful in encouraging a black or mixed identity in their children were often part of a network of interracial families and 'had abandoned *full* membership of the white group' (Wilson 1987, p. ix, original emphasis). Echoing the theme of changing social locations, Nick Banks (1996), a clinical psychologist, describes the treatment of sixteen young (seventeen to twenty-three years old) lone white mothers of mixed-parentage children in therapy. Emerging themes included social isolation from both black and white communities, possible loss of contact with the mother's birth family due to abandonment and rejection, and stigma.

More recent work has pointed to the embeddedness of white mothers within the black Caribbean community. France Winndance Twine's (2004) ethnographic research involving lone and partnered mothers in interracial families provided insight into the way that contact with black friends can be significant in terms of enhancing mothers' 'racial literacy', which is linked to their attempts to protect their children against the influence of racism. Interestingly, Twine (2010) reported that married mothers experienced higher levels of social isolation and attended fewer social events than those who were lone parents, which suggests that contrary to fears about isolation, lone mothers' activities could even put them at an advantage in terms of social contact.

Another ethnographic study by Elaine Bauer (2010) considered the experiences of thirty-four mixed-couple families of whom nineteen comprised a white British female and an African-Caribbean male. She found: 'Among the mixed families themselves, there has been an ongoing dynamic process of modification involving family conflict, rejection, violence, adaptation, accommodation and innovation/creativity in order to survive as families and kindreds' (Bauer 2010, p. 246). Lisa McKenzie's (2010) ethnographic study of the Nottingham council estate St Ann's is also relevant. She interviewed thirty-five lone and partnered mothers of mixed-parentage children and found that the women were acutely aware of stigma and judgement from those outside of the estate because they were living on a council estate, claiming benefits and were mothers to mixed-parentage children. This led them to look 'inwards' to the estate for local inclusion. McKenzie (2010) argues that on the estate Caribbean culture was valued and mixing was viewed positively, therefore being a mother of mixed-parentage children was a source of status. Focusing specifically on lone mothers of children of mixed racial and ethnic parentage, Caballero and Edwards (2010) interviewed ten lone mothers in south-west England and compared their experiences to mothers of children from mixed racial and ethnic backgrounds in the 1960s using the secondary analysis of qualitative interviews. The findings identify areas both of continuity and change in social reactions and support networks, with friendships highlighted as important for both samples.

In recent years technological advances have made communication across space easier and more affordable, with technology such as Skype, social networking (such as Facebook), as well as more affordable air travel. These provide greater opportunity for family members living apart to connect on a more regular basis. There has also been a growth in the online information and support available for interracial families, with organizations such as People in Harmony and Intermix, providing online information and support that families and individuals can access.

While the review of the existing literature has highlighted key themes including marginalization, stigma from wider society and integration into Caribbean networks, in many of the studies it is difficult to disaggregate the experiences of lone and partnered mothers. This paper aims to contribute to the existing literature by providing an in-depth discussion of the informal support networks utilized by lone white mothers of mixed-parentage children and to employ the concept of social capital to illuminate the value of the different elements of support that are available.

Methodology

This paper draws on interviews with thirty lone white mothers of mixed-parentage children conducted between March 2004 and January 2005. Interviewees were recruited from a variety of sources including support groups for black and interracial families ($n = 11$), a regional multiple heritage service ($n = 7$), social services ($n = 2$), support groups for lone parents ($n=4$), an NSPCC family support service ($n=2$), a regional race relations unit ($n=1$), an agency assisting lone parents to find employment ($n=1$) and snowballing ($n=2$). The interviews began using a social network map (Tracy and Whittaker 1990). This is a visual representation of a circle divided into a number of segments in order to gain information about social networks in each area (e.g. friends, neighbours, clubs/organizations/ church, formal services). In-depth interviews were chosen as the main research method in order to allow participants time and space to discuss their experiences from their own point of view (Oakley 1998) and to allow the flexibility to follow up what interviewees considered to be important. Interview topics included the following: people found to be most helpful and supportive; anyone with whom the relationship is stressful or difficult; practices employed to promote positive identity development; experiences of racism; and areas in which mothers would like more support. All interviews were conducted face-to-face. They ranged from fifty minutes to three and a half hours in length and were tape-recorded with the permission of the interviewee.

Each interview was transcribed in full and research notes were typed up. All names and potentially identifiable details were changed to protect anonymity. Framework analysis was used to analyse the qualitative data. This is a systematic approach to analysing qualitative data that involves five key stages: familiarization; identifying a thematic framework; indexing; charting; and interpretation (see Ritchie and Spencer 1994). The software package Atlas.ti was used to assist with managing the data.

Mothers participating in the study were drawn from a range of geographical locations including London, Manchester, Nottingham, Brighton, Bristol, Sheffield, Surrey, Hertfordshire and East Sussex. Interviewees ranged from twenty to forty-nine years old, with the mean age being thirty-six. The majority of mothers ($n=22$) were single and had never been married, while seven were divorced and one was separated. In terms of employment, sixteen mothers held a paid job while fourteen mothers did not. Occupations included receptionist, food preparation, customer service, administrator, manager for a voluntary organization, counsellor, social worker and small business owner.

To give some indication of level of income, the mothers were asked if they were currently living on state benefits. A majority of twenty-three mothers were currently receiving benefits, while seven were not. Almost half of the sample ($n=14$) lived in local authority rented accommodation while eight mothers owned their own homes and five rented their homes privately. In addition to this, one mother lived in a housing cooperative, one lived with her parents and one lived with a relative for whom she was the full-time carer.

Mothers in the study had between one and five children, with one or two being most common. Mothers had children aged from a few months to twenty years, with the majority aged between four and fifteen years. Prior to the interview, demographic information was collected using a brief profile questionnaire. Using the 2001 census categories, the majority of children ($n = 37$) were described as 'Mixed White and Black Caribbean' by their mothers. Following this eleven children were categorized as 'Mixed White and Black African', four as 'Mixed White and Asian' and six as 'Any Other Mixed Background'. Finally, three children were described as white (two mothers had white children as well as mixed-parentage children). Having outlined the methodology employed, this paper moves on to consider the key findings in different areas of mothers' support networks. The discussion of the findings begins by looking at the support provided by friends, before moving on to explore the relationship with the mother's extended family, children's father's, the paternal family and support groups.

Friends

The role of friends is at the forefront of debates around individualization and transformation of intimacy (Pahl and Pevalin 2005), where it is argued that people are now less tied into old patterns of obligation and family ties. The literature on friendship theory illustrates that friendships are not static but that life events such as becoming a mother, moving house, going to university and marital or relationship breakdown can influence friendship networks and social capital (Reynolds 2007). Friendships are also influenced by ethnicity. For example, Tracey Reynolds (2007) explored the friendship networks of Caribbean young people in Britain and found that while they had friends across diverse ethnic groups, their closest friends tended to share their ethnic background. This was partly because friends of the same ethnic background provided a source of trust, understanding and emotional support that acted as a buffer to social exclusion and racial discrimination within wider society (Reynolds 2007).

When asked who had been most helpful and supportive to them in their task of parenting, most mothers in the present study named female friends. Friends were found to be a source of emotional support and often also provided practical assistance, such as picking up children from school. Illustrating the importance of friends, one mother, Meg, explained: 'I always keep my friends close round me.' Another mother, Miriam, commented that her friendship network was 'a really important part of my decision to have a child by myself.' Judy described her friends as 'like a second family', suggesting that she and her friends share the closeness and intimacy of people born into the same kinship group. Furthermore, some mothers explained how friends provided a listening ear, allowing them to talk about personal problems or concerns. A number of mothers highlighted the ethnic diversity of their friendship groups and their narratives suggested that they saw this as related to having mixed-parentage children. For example, Bethany, a thirty-one-year-old mother who lived in a diverse area, said: 'I've only got like a couple of white friends and the rest are themselves Afro-Caribbean, Pakistani or Arabic, you know.' A minority of mothers described how some friendships with former white friends had been lost as a result of racist attitudes. For example, Paula, a twenty-eight-year-old mother of three children, said that a lot of her white friends 'disowned' her when she and her children's father began their relationship. Throughout their relationship, Paula and her ex-partner spent more time with his friends. She said that she is pleased that these friendships have been maintained since the relationship broke down and she became a lone parent.

A number of mothers spoke about black friends being an important source of support. For example, Leanne, a thirty-two-year-old mother of three children, talked about her strong friendships with people from African-Caribbean backgrounds and she argued that they acted as 'role models' for her children. Through such friendships she was also able to gain access to Caribbean culture, which she felt was very important to pass on to her children. For example, she was being taught to cook Caribbean food by her next-door neighbour and was also learning about black history. At the time of the interview she talked about her plans to set up a business selling black hair products. Another mother, Denise (aged thirty-two) explained that she was concerned when she came home to find her daughter scrubbing herself with a white bar of soap after being called racist names at school. She described how advice from an older female friend who was like a grandmother to her children provided support in this situation. It could be suggested that such friendships were particularly important because they have the potential to provide a different kind of support to that provided by the white extended family. For example, Denise had brought her children black dolls in order to try to strengthen their self-concept in light of the racism they had experienced. However, her parents could not understand why Denise bought her children black dolls, and accused her of trying to deny the white side of their heritage. This suggests that some mothers received a particular kind of support and understanding from black friends that was valuable to them in their role as mothers of mixed-parentage children. Interestingly, another mother in the study described how Denise, in turn, had been particularly helpful and supportive to her in terms of teaching her how to braid her daughter's hair.

Many mothers in the study explained that they found other white mothers of mixed-parentage children to be particularly supportive because they gave non-judgemental support and empathy. As Bethany explains:

Having someone in your situation ... You know that you can talk with so that you know if you're feeling down about something and you find out that same person's feeling down about that same situation, it makes you feel a bit better.

Mothers described that situations they may feel 'down about' included negotiating racist attitudes directed at their children, as well as social disapproval directed at themselves (Harman 2010). Caballero and Edwards (2010) compared the experiences of interracial families in 1960s and the present day and similarly pointed to the important role of informal networks of friends in the same situation among both samples. However, not all mothers in the present study held friendships with other lone mothers. Amanda, a twenty-six-year-old mother of two, explained that she would like to have friendships with other mothers in a similar situation to her:

I don't really know of any other lone white mothers of mixed heritage children, and that would be quite nice to have, even just a pen friend, that was in the same situation as me, that would be nice. You know because although I do have friends who have got mixed heritage children, they're not quite in the same situation as me because they've got their partners around. And their children also have got their fathers around to draw a positive image from. And it would be nice for me to have support from somebody who was in exactly the situation that I was in.

Lone parenthood acted as a further reference point with regard to who mothers perceived to be in the same situation as them. Many mothers suggested that not having the child's father in the home offered a distinct set of experiences, including the need for additional resources to strengthen the child's ethnic identity. In addition, some mothers described that they perceived they were viewed with suspicion on attending social events attended by mixed couples – they felt that they were, on occasion, seen as a sexual threat because they were single.

The close friendships among lone white mothers of mixed-parentage children documented here could be seen as bonding social capital. Mothers perceived that there were shared experiences and somewhat of a shared identity as a result of mothering mixed-parentage children. This related to positively valuing mixing across ethnic boundaries and being aware of the effects of racism. These friendships were highlighted as particularly valuable for empathy, advice and non-judgemental support.

Family

After friends, mothers' own mothers were identified as providing a considerable amount of support. Interestingly, Pahl and Pevalin (2005) argue that the distinction between friends and family is not clear-cut – many people choose their friends from among their kin and the likelihood of doing so increases with age. Amy, a twenty-nine-year-old mother, described her appreciation at the support she had received from her mother:

> From day one she's always been there for me, you know throughout my pregnancy, she was there when I gave birth...and she was the person who brought me back from the hospital and helped me with dealing with sleepless nights and just looked after me, at a time when I really desperately needed somebody to do that.

When the interview took place, Amy was living with her mother and stepfather and felt that this had sheltered her from the most difficult aspects of being a lone parent, which she perceived to be loneliness and financial difficulties. Previous research concerning the experience of lone mothers has also emphasized the importance of support provided by a lone mother's own mother (Dearlove 1999; Ghate and Hazel 2002). According to Dearlove (1999), the availability of support from the lone mother's mother is crucial in influencing whether she is lone or alone.

In the present study, family contact was often felt to be very important despite long distances between relatives. Contact was made by phone and visits to and from family members were considered important. However, not all mothers had supportive relationships with their families. For example, referring to difficult relationships with some members of her extended family, Toni, a twenty-year-old mother of two, said: 'It's like the old thing "it takes a village to raise a child", but the village doesn't want to help if you have a child with someone of a different race.'

As reported in more detail elsewhere (Harman 2010), some mothers were negotiating overtly racist views of family members, including in more severe cases, being 'disowned' by members of their family. For example, Leanne, a thirty-two-year-old mother of three, described her experience:

> I met my eldest son's Dad and I started a relationship with him, much against my parent's will. I was actually disowned from my

parents, from a lot of people actually...It was really quite lonely, and "oh you nigger lover" and lots of horrible names I was called. My Mum obviously didn't want me to keep my son under any circumstances...I'm the only daughter so for my Dad it just shattered his whole dreams. It was just not what he wanted.

Leanne now has contact with her mother, who has expressed regret at the sentiments she expressed when Leanne was pregnant. However, Leanne questions whether her father's attitudes have really changed and contact with him is occasional and strained. In some cases disapproval softens when the child arrives and relationships are rebuilt over time, but in others relationships remain difficult or non-existent (Harman 2010).

Within the literature on social capital, bonding capital is understood as relationships reinforcing identities, trust and values within homogenous groups (Putnam 2000). As bonding capital involves people with similar backgrounds and shared norms and values, this has the capacity to exclude as well as to include (Bruegel 2005). Following this argument, exclusion from white familial or friendship groups could be seen as a result of having broken one of the norms and values of the network – to engage in mono-ethnic intimate relationships. The findings also show that it is possible for attitudes to change over time.

Besides the influence of racism in severing aspects of mothers' support networks that may otherwise have been available, there were also other reasons as to why some families could offer more limited or no support. For example, one mother explained that she had been taken into care as a child and that this had had implications for contact with her family. A small number of mothers explained that one or both of their parents had passed away and some mothers explained that their parents were elderly and needed considerable support themselves, which meant that they were primarily the providers rather than recipients of support.

Contact with the child's father

In many cases, contact with the child's father was found to be the most stressful part of the mother's social network. However, the majority of fathers had some form of contact with their children at the time of the interview and just over half were described as having regular contact. The sample showed considerable diversity regarding the nature and frequency of contact with children's fathers. Toni explained that she had a good relationship with her children's father: 'He comes round after work maybe twice a week and I take the kids to his mum's on Saturday and he comes round. Sometimes he comes for dinner on Sunday and things like that.'

In some cases where fathers now had regular contact, the level of contact had increased over time. Some mothers had received formal support in their relationship with their ex-partner, including mediation or supervised visits.

Where fathers were described as having irregular or occasional contact with their children, this was often found to be very stressful. For example, Jenny, a thirty-five-year-old mother of two, described the stress caused by the infrequent contact that her children have with their father:

> Janet and Matthew probably see their dad nearly two or three times a year, if that . . . the last time he was meant to have them [was] in July and he didn't show up anyway. And he didn't pick up the phone to say why, he didn't pick up the phone to apologise, he just didn't turn up. He's turned up at two o'clock in the morning before to pick up his children when he should have been there at three o'clock in the afternoon . . . but because my kids had been so looking forward to see their dad and going, I wasn't going to prevent them, although I did say to him afterwards "Don't ever turn up at that time again otherwise I refuse to let my children go." . . . It hurts me as a mother when I see my children hurting, when I see my children sobbing and crying, and Matthew . . . it's like it's my fault when his daddy doesn't come.

For Jenny, such episodes had been extremely distressing because she had been left to explain to her children why their father had not arrived without knowing the reason herself and had had to deal with their disappointment. Of the fathers not currently in contact with their children at the time of the interview, there were various reasons and situations surrounding this, including difficult relationships between parents, residence in other countries and never having been involved in the child's life from the beginning. For example, Amanda explained that she had met her son's father in a nightclub and they had had a brief relationship:

> He left when I was five weeks pregnant and that's the last I saw of him. He'd wanted me to have an abortion, and he lives in [another city], so I've not sort of bumped into him or anything. He hasn't contacted me and I haven't contacted him. So he doesn't know whether I've had a boy or a girl or anything.

The considerable diversity in contact with children's fathers cautions against making generalizations or stereotypes about their absence or otherwise. Caballero and Edwards (2010) similarly found variability in levels of contact with fathers among the ten lone mothers that they interviewed. While mothers in the present study generally positioned children's fathers as outside of their own support network, the frequency of contact and the nature of the relationship were salient factors contributing to mothers' experience of parenting, their stress levels and their concerns about their children's ethnic identity development. Without the child's father resident in the home, contact with the father's family often took on greater significance.

Contact with extended family on the father's side

It was found that children had some contact with the extended family on the father's side in about three-quarters of cases. Some mothers described their efforts to maintain relationships between themselves and the father's family when the relationship ended. For example, Jaclyn, a thirty-eight-year-old mother, said:

That was just one thing I was very strong about and then they carried on when we split up, I kept contact with his mum. I made sure that she knew that I wouldn't just disappear with the kids that she'd still see her grandchildren 'cos she was very close to them. So I was keen to keep that connection going and worked hard to do it.

Contact with the extended family was seen as important for giving children a sense of their paternal cultural heritage and assisting their ethnic identity development. Rebecca, a forty-year-old mother of two, spoke positively about contact with her children's grandmother:

It's great that they get to see their grandmother when she comes over from Nigeria and that all sort of seems very normal that she'll be wearing her African dress and stuff like that. You know I'm pleased we've been able to maintain that but I think if we'd been together they would have had that whole richness which they really don't have.

Rebecca suggested that contact with her children's grandmother was particularly important as her children did not have regular contact with their father and they lived in a mainly white area. However, because the grandmother lived in Nigeria this meant limited oppor-tunities for contact, with visits about once per year. Previous research has highlighted that some minority ethnic families may have limited contact with grandparents due to residence in different countries (Barn et al. 2006). The present study suggests that this is also a consideration for some lone mothers of mixed-parentage children; however, despite distance, contact was often viewed as a central link to the children's heritage.

Mothers who did not have contact from the black family remarked upon the perceived lack of input and some mothers expressed frustration that they were being left without adequate support. The phrase 'I can only do so much' was repeated across a number of interviews, expressing the feeling that mothers were already coping with a lot in bringing up their children as a lone parent, without the added pressure of providing awareness and appreciation of the paternal heritage – a task that some mothers felt they were unqualified to do on their own. Illustrating this, Jenny explained:

> I tried my hardest as a parent to raise my children and show them love, to discipline them, to guide them, to support them. But I have very little knowledge of black history and black culture and black heritage . . . Juliana [Jenny's friend of African-Caribbean heritage] is very up on that and you know she can give me information but this is the thing, I feel that I'm very numb. I go to work, I look after the house, I take my children to all these different activities, we go to church, I'm there as a mother as well, there's only so much I could do in my time with the hours of the day that I have and with my own capabilities . . . So it's not through lack of wanting to or wishing to . . . I would like so much that my children would be able to have an outside input. I mean for instance if I was still with their father or even if I wasn't but he had a significant part in their lives and if they spent time with his family they probably would get that influence.

As previous research has suggested (Ali 2003; Twine 2004, 2010), black and minority ethnic friends were often seen as a valuable source of cultural and anti-racist information. It could be argued that relationships between mothers and members of the paternal family constitute a form of bridging social capital – outward-looking relationships where trust is developed between members of different social groups. The findings suggested that mothers perceived these relationships as being able to provide a 'different type' of support than that experienced from the white extended family. Mothers connected contact with the paternal family and black friends with strengthening children's self-concept, their ethnic identity and by extension their ability to cope with racism. However, not all mothers had regular supportive contact with the child's father or his family. In the absence of the father and his family, support groups were sometimes accessed for help.

Support groups

A relatively high proportion of mothers within the sample had used a support group, either for lone parents, for black and interracial families or directed towards interracial families and individuals specifically. This is likely to be related to the recruitment method for the study, which used, as one tool, advertisements placed in the newsletters of these groups. One motivating factor for joining a support group was found to be the opportunity to meet people in a similar situation. This provided the potential for informal discussion about experiences and concerns. On learning about a group in her local area, Julie (aged forty-five) said: 'It was very reassuring to know there was something like that for us. Yeah, it was really quite exciting to hear of it.' Mothers explained that becoming actively involved in a support group had increased their self-esteem as well as providing social connections. In addition to receiving support, some mothers experienced opportunities for involvement as many semi-formal services rely on volunteers to keep running (Ghate and Hazel 2002). For example, two young parents living in a diverse area described how they had joined a support group for lone parents. Over time, as a result of their participation and ideas, they were asked to help to run a parenting programme specifically for younger parents. Lori, a twenty-four-year-old mother, explained: 'We do talk about racial issues that happen within the community. And like "Never guess what happened the other day, this happened." And someone was like "What?" and we just talk about it and discuss it, kind of thing.'

Support groups were perceived by their members as less rigid and fixed than formal services, giving mothers the scope to discuss issues of concern to them. As Heather (aged thirty-two) explained: 'It's non-judgemental, and plus they can identify with your experiences.' As highlighted by Boushel (1996), mothers also suggested that groups were providing support in relation to racism. For example, Jasmine (aged thirty-eight) described how her local group had assisted her when she heard that the secondary school that her daughter had been allocated to had a problem with racism. Through this group she was able to access letters from other parents whose children had experienced racism at this school, which acted as supporting evidence for her appeal against the school place decision.

While some mothers had continued to be active members of support groups, others found that contact had reduced over time. Julie said that support groups for black and interracial families may be more useful for those who do not have minority ethnic friends as part of their informal networks. Even where mothers felt that regular participation in the activities of support groups was not for them, they often continued to have some marginal contact, for example receiving newsletters, which may be useful to point them to other activities or sources of support.

Contact with support groups, it could be argued, offers mothers the opportunity to extend both their bonding capital, by providing opportunities to meet other white mothers in interracial families, and also their bridging capital, by increasing the potential to make friends from minority ethnic backgrounds. Additionally, support groups could potentially provide linking capital through giving mothers access to resources and increased power to deal with racism. Given their potential value to lone white mothers of mixed-parentage children, it is important that such groups receive adequate funding in order to allow them to reach out to families. For example, online resources provide an opportunity for mothers living in mainly white rural areas to make contact with others in a similar situation.

Discussion and conclusion

With a considerable proportion of mixed-parentage children in Britain living in lone-parent families (Platt 2009), there is a need for an increased understanding of the support networks available to this specific group. In each of the areas explored in this paper – friends, family, contact with the children's father and his family and support groups – considerable diversity was evident among the experiences of the mothers in the sample. However, some key themes can be highlighted. Although the salience of ethnicity has often been neglected when white people are researched (Frankenberg 1993; Byrne 2006), the findings suggest that ethnicity plays an important role in shaping the social networks of white mothers of mixed-parentage children. Mothers' own identity, concern for the development of their children's identity and lone parenthood influenced their support networks in significant ways. The interviews suggested that for some mothers, entering into an interracial relationship or having mixed-parentage children led to a loss of some friendships or family relationships due to the effects of racism. As well as mothers' support networks being constrained in this way, their experiences provided motivation to reach out to people who they felt were supportive of their parenting. In the USA, Hill and Thomas (2000, p. 198) similarly highlight that women in interracial partnerships 'intentionally create and nurture communities of relationships in which they can shape their racial identities with support apart from the constraints of racism.'

Mothers' parenting experiences led to an impetus to enlarge their support networks in particular directions, for example through support groups, friendships with people from minority ethnic back-grounds and other interracial families. Friendships are not static across the life course but are influenced by life events such as becoming a mother (Reynolds 2007). Furthermore, the literature on family and friendship formation and maintenance indicates that people operate a discerning approach regarding the family and friendship relationships that they nurture, based around shared values, common interests and similarities (Pahl and Pevalin 2005). The findings suggest that shared concerns and perceived emotional connectedness are key to understanding social capital of lone white mothers of mixed-parentage children. Mothers' impetus to extend their social network was also related to lone parenthood and a perception of the need to find people and resources outside the household to support the children's identity development. Previous research has highlighted the way in which networks are comprised of 'different strokes from different folks', whereby friends (in particular women) are likely to provide emotional support and companionship, while parents are more likely to provide financial aid and services (Wellman and Wortley 1990). Findings from the present study suggest that other white mothers of mixed-parentage children, black friends and the black extended family were felt to offer different types of support than that experienced from the white extended family. In particular, they were seen to be able to offer more support in terms of racial and cultural identity development and dealing with racism. Some mothers described how they were 'working hard' to maintain relationships with members of the paternal family because they thought that they would be beneficial to their children throughout their life. This echoes Bourdieu's (1987) assertion that mothers are often investing in social capital for their children, but demonstrates how this can be linked to ethnicity as well as social class.

Through in-depth qualitative interviews with thirty mothers, this paper has explored mothers' perceptions of their informal support networks. The analysis has suggested that racism and identity influence mothers' support networks, both acting as a constraining force as well as providing opportunities and impetuses for pursuing contact that mothers felt would support their parenting. The findings highlight the patterns of inclusion and exclusion that influence the social capital of lone white mothers of mixed-parentage children.

Acknowledgements

The author would like to thank the research participants. This research was funded by the Economic and Social Research Council (Award no. PTA033200200051).

References

ALI, SUKI 2003 *Mixed-Race, Post-Race: Gender, New Ethnicities and Cultural Practices*, Oxford: Berg
ATTREE, PAMELA 2005 'Parenting support in the context of poverty: a meta-synthesis of the qualitative evidence', *Health and Social Care in the Community*, vol. 13, no. 4, pp. 330–7
BANKS, NICK 1996 'Young single white mothers with black children in therapy', *Clinical Child Psychology and Psychiatry*, vol. 1, no. 1, pp. 19–28
BARN, RAVINDER 1999 'White mothers, mixed-parentage children and child welfare', *British Journal of Social Work*, vol. 29, no. 2, pp. 269–84

BARN, RAVINDER *et al.* 2006 *Parenting in Multi-Racial Britain*, London: National Children's Bureau

BARNES, JACQUELINE 2007 *Down our Way: The Relevance of Neighbourhoods for Parenting and Child Development*, Chichester: John Wiley and Sons

BAUER, ELAINE 2010 *The Creolisation of London Kinship: Mixed African-Caribbean and White British Extended Families, 1950–2003*, Amsterdam: Amsterdam University Press

BOURDIEU, PIERRE 1987 'The forms of capital', in John G. Richardson (ed.), *Handbook of Theory and Research for the Sociology of Education*, New York: Greenwood Press, pp. 241–58

BOUSHEL, MARGARET 1996 'Vulnerable multiracial families and early years services: concerns, challenges and opportunities', *Children and Society*, vol. 10, no. 4, pp. 305–16

BRUEGEL, IRENE 2005 'Social capital and feminist critique', in Jane Franklin (ed.), *Women and Social Capital, Working Paper No. 12*, London: South Bank University, Families and Social Capital ESRC Research Group, pp. 4–17

BYRNE, BRIDGET 2006 *White Lives: The Interplay of 'Race', Class and Gender in Everyday Life*, Abingdon: Routledge

CABALLERO, CHAMION and EDWARDS, ROSALIND 2010 *Lone Mothers of Mixed Racial and Ethnic Children: Then and Now*, London: Runnymede Trust

DEARLOVE, JOSEPHINE 1999 'Lone or alone? A qualitative study of lone mothers on low incomes with reference to support in their everyday lives', PhD thesis, University of Warwick

EDWARDS, ROSALIND, FRANKLIN, JANE and HOLLAND, JANET 2003 *Families and Social Capital: Exploring the Issues,* Working Paper No. 1, London: South Bank University, Families and Social Capital ESRC Research Group

FRANKENBERG, RUTH 1993 *The Social Construction of Whiteness: White Women, Race Matters*, London: Routledge

GARDNER, RUTH 2003 *Supporting Families: Child Protection in the Community*, Chichester: Wiley

GHATE, DEBORAH and HAZEL, NEAL 2002 *Parenting in Poor Environments: Stress, Support and Coping*, London: Jessica Kingsley Publishers

HALPERN, DAVID 2005 *Social Capital*, Cambridge: Polity Press

HARMAN, VICKI 2010 'Experiences of racism and the changing nature of white privilege among lone white mothers of mixed-parentage children in the UK', *Ethnic and Racial Studies*, vol. 33, no. 3, pp. 176–94

HILL, MIRIAM and VOLKER, THOMAS 2000 'Strategies for racial identity development: narratives of black and white women in interracial partner relationships', *Family Relations*, vol. 49, no. 2, pp. 193–200

MCKENZIE, LISA 2010 'Finding value on a council estate: complex lives, motherhood, and exclusion', PhD thesis, University of Nottingham

OAKLEY, ANN 1998 'Gender, methodology and people's ways of knowing: some problems with feminism and the paradigm debate in social science', *Sociology*, vol. 32, no. 4, pp. 707–31

OWEN, CHARLIE 2005 'Looking at numbers and projections: making sense of the census and emerging trends', in Toyin Okitikpi (ed.), *Working with Children of Mixed Parentage*, Dorset: Russell House Publishing, pp. 10–26

PAHL, RAY and PEVALIN, D. 2005 'Between family and friends: a longitudinal study of friendship choice', *The British Journal of Sociology*, vol. 56, no. 3, pp. 433–50

PLATT, LUCINDA 2009 *Ethnicity and Family: Relationships within and between Ethnic Groups: An Analysis Using the Labour Force Survey*, London: Equality and Human Rights Commission

PUTNAM, ROBERT 1995 'Bowling alone: America's declining social capital', *Journal of Democracy*, vol. 6, no. 1, pp. 65–78

——— 2000 *Bowling Alone: The Collapse and Revival of American Community*, New York: Simon and Schuster Paperbacks

———— 2007 'E Pluribus Unum: diversity and community in the twenty-first century: the 2006 Johan Skytte Prize lecture', *Scandinavian Political Studies*, vol. 30, no. 2, pp. 137–74

REYNOLDS, TRACEY 2007 'Friendship networks, social capital and ethnic identity: researching the perspectives of Caribbean young people in Britain', *Journal of Youth Studies*, vol. 10, no. 4, pp. 383–98

———— 2010 'Editorial introduction: young people, social capital and ethnicity', *Ethnic and Racial Studies*, vol. 33, no. 5, pp. 749–60

RITCHIE, JANE and SPENCER, LIZ 1994 'Qualitative data analysis for applied policy research', in Alan Bryman and Bob Burgess (eds), *Analysing Qualitative Data*, London: Routledge, pp. 173–94

ROWLINGSON, KAREN and MCKAY, STEPHEN 2002 *Lone Parent Families: Gender, Class and State*, Harlow: Prentice Hall

TRACY, ELIZABETH and WHITTAKER, JAMES 1990 'The social network map: assessing social support in clinical practice', *Families in Society*, vol. 71, no. 8, pp. 461–70

TWINE, FRANCE WINDDANCE 2004 'A white side of black Britain: the concept of racial literacy', *Ethnic and Racial Studies*, vol. 27, no. 6, pp. 878–907

———— 2010 *A White Side of Black Britain: Interracial Intimacy and Racial Literacy*, Durham, NC: Duke University Press

WELLMAN, BARRY and WORTLEY, SCOT 1990 'Different strokes from different folks: community ties and social support', *American Journal of Sociology*, vol. 96, no. 3, pp. 558–88

WILSON, ANN 1981 'In between: the mother in the interracial family', *New Community*, vol. 9, no. 2, pp. 208–15

———— 1987 *Mixed Race Children: A Study of Identity*, London: Allen and Unwin

Narratives from a Nottingham council estate: a story of white working-class mothers with mixed-race children

Lisa McKenzie

Abstract

This paper introduces a group of white working-class women living on a council estate in the UK drawing on an ethnographic study conducted between 2005 and 2009, examining the impact of class inequality and a stigmatized living space in an ethnically diverse urban neighbourhood. All of the women are mothers and have mixed-race children; they reside on the St Ann's estate in Nottingham, an inner-city neighbourhood that has been subject to poor housing, poverty and unemployment for many generations. The women who live on this estate say that they suffer from negative stereotypes and stigmatization because of the notoriety of the estate, because they are working class and because they have had sexual relationships with black men. However, there is a sense of connectedness to the estate and there are strong cultural meanings that are heavily influenced by the West Indian community. This paper then highlights the importance of place when focusing upon families, class inequality and intercultural relationships.

Introduction

This paper introduces a group of white working-class women living on a council estate (public housing) in the UK drawing on an ethnographic study conducted between 2005 and 2009, examining the impact of class inequality and a stigmatized living space in an ethnically diverse urban neighbourhood. All of the women are mothers and have mixed-race children; they reside on the St Ann's estate in Nottingham, an inner-city neighbourhood that has been subject to poor housing, poverty and unemployment for many generations (Coates and Silburn 1970; Johns 2002). The women who live on this estate say that they suffer from negative stereotypes and stigmatization because of the notoriety of the estate, because they are working class and because they have had sexual relationships with black men.

In recent years there has been a disproportionate amount of moral panic, fear and political gesturing aimed at a specific section of the British working class. Those who live in social housing, have irregular and poorly paid employment and subsequently rely on welfare benefits are often referenced within the 'underclass' discourse (Lister 1996; Levitas 2005; Welshman 2006). However, this moral outrage has been particularly vengeful in relation to council estate residents and, more specifically, those mothers who live on them with their children. It seems that the political classes from all parties have agreed that our British council estates are severe social problems. As the Conservative Party – and now coalition government – constantly reminds us, Britain is broken and its council estates 'are broken ghettos'; this has led to its current position that there are 120,000 specific 'troubled families' reliant upon welfare benefits and social housing (Duncan-Smith 2008; West 2009; Riddell 2010). There has been a particular preoccupation with the notion that the broken and troubled families are specifically located on the many council estates in Britain and the names of some of these estates have become shorthand for expressing everything that is wrong and loathsome about British society (Lawler 2003; Skeggs 2004; Rogaly and Taylor 2009). The St Ann's estate in Nottingham is an example of how stigmatized neighbourhoods and their residents have become inextricably linked: as many residents note, you do not simply reside within St Ann's, you *are* St Ann's. The women who have taken part in this research acknowledge the stigmatization of 'being St Ann's' but also acknowledge that they have 'other crosses to bear': they have had sexual relationships with black men and their children are mixed-race, which, they say, further stigmatizes them as 'rough and ready' outside of the estate.

However, while the political and media debate paints a bleakly homogenous landscape of social alienation and abandonment of hope in poorer neighbourhoods, or of segregated inner-city communities embattled and suffering at the hands of 'mass immigration', the people who live on this estate in Nottingham tell of a far more complexly textured life. They speak of adaptation, cooperation and a reflexive awareness of their lives. Their accounts are inflected with recognition of heterogeneity and a sense of positive as well as negative aspects of estate life.

This paper offers an account of understanding how specific neighbourhoods become devalued, and how families become stigma-tized. In this case in Nottingham, the process of stigmatization is specifically related to being council estate mothers and white women who have had sexual relationships with black men, and are consequently mothers to mixed-race children. Nevertheless, and without neglecting the often harsh social realities families who live in poor neighbourhoods face, the mothers on this estate have found respect and value at a local level, from their relationships with the West Indian community and their highly recognized local status of motherhood.

The article examines how Pierre Bourdieu's (1986, 1990, 1999) thesis relating to the poorest and most stigmatized neighbourhoods that have little institutional capital – that is, employment, skills and education, the very resources that allow groups, individuals and communities a wider societal value – can be used in understanding how socially excluded neighbourhoods find respect, value and community within their local neighbourhoods. The paper argues that those communities who are denied access to these valuable resources do not simply sit down and accept their fate, but instead engage in a local system that gives value to individuals and the community, based upon local networks and a shared cultural understanding of how the estate works. The women in Nottingham who have taken part in this study invest in this local value system and look to the resources within to feel valued and valuable, even when those local resources are often mis-recognized, dis-respected or are simply invisible to 'others'. This paper explores the consequences of class inequality for working-class women living in an ethnically diverse urban neighbourhood – thus, raising important questions about class and race in Britain, the consequences of becoming stigmatized, and how communities, families and individuals manage those issues relating to class inequality.

Methodology in a local neighbourhood

The St Ann's estate is one of the poorest 10 per cent of neighbourhoods in the UK, and has been identified officially as 'socially excluded' (ONS 2007). Over decades, the neighbourhood has been subject to a number of harsh social realities: unemployment and low pay, and lack of decent housing and good education (Coates and Silburn 1970, 1980; Johns 2002). Locally, it has become stigmatized with a reputation as a place to avoid, supposedly full of crime and drugs, single mums and benefit claimants. The neighbourhood also has a long history as the place where the poorest and migrant workers have resided in Nottingham; people from Ireland, the West Indies, Italy, Poland and South East Asia have been documented as living in St Ann's since the early 1950s (Coates and Silburn 1970; Johns 2002; Solomos 2003). The neighbourhood has always been in flux, with people moving in and then, as they become more financially secure, often moving out. However, the West Indian and especially Jamaican populations who arrived from the 1950s have stayed constant, creating homes, families and communities.

The research focused on a group of thirty-five women living on the St Ann's council estate in Nottingham, who are white and are mothers to mixed-race children. The study aimed to examine how this group of women find value for themselves and their families when their estate and its residents are often represented as spaces and people of no or little value. The women varied in age, with the youngest a nineteen-year-old mother with a six-week-old daughter, and the eldest a fifty-six-year-old mother with eight children and numerous grandchildren and great-grandchildren. All of the children's fathers were African-Caribbean or of African-Caribbean descent, usually second- or third-generation migrant families predominantly coming from Jamaica in the late 1950s and early 1960s. The women referred to themselves as 'white English, Irish or Scottish'. They preferred to call their children 'mixed-race' rather than 'dual heritage', which they thought sounded 'too American', and the women with older children said they were 'tired of it' (the description of their children) being changed every few years. Furthermore, they also objected to 'dual heritage' because it had become the preferred term used by teachers at the local schools, and the women felt that neither they nor their children had been consulted by anyone in authority over which terms to use to describe them.

It is important that I discuss my own connection to the neighbour-hood. I undertook the research, mapped the neighbourhood and interpreted the findings, but at the same time I am also a long-term resident of this estate, having lived in St Ann's for more than twenty years with my own family. Therefore, the ethnographic methodology used for the study did not present the usual challenges of access and familiarity: I was already part of the local community; my own children had attended the local schools and youth clubs; and, as a white working-class woman and mother of mixed-race children who also had only lived on council estates, there was a commonality between the women and myself. Nevertheless, it would be wrong to underestimate not only the ease but also the difficulties within the relationships I formed with the women and their families. At times, my positioning as resident and researcher was extremely strained; the unfair and negative representations of the women in this community often left them very defensive and since I also lived there, the women knew that I was aware of the stereotypes about the neighbourhood. Consequently, there were initial concerns about how I might use my local knowledge and whether it would add to the negative portrayal of the estate and their families. The insider status I held was often difficult to negotiate within the research process and I cannot deny that my own position swings – from valueless St Ann's resident to valuable academic researcher.

Stigmatization

Negative and mean representations of poor working-class people and the places where they live are widespread in the UK and have been well documented in the work of Skeggs (1997, 2004, 2009), Nayak (2009), Lawler (2005), Reay (2000, 2002, 2004), Haylett (2000, 2001), Munt (2000) and Sibley (1995). Lawler (2008, p. 133) argues that working-class people are rarely named as class subjects but are often known and reproduced as 'disgusting subjects', usually through descriptions of bodies and clothing, which are used as shorthand for stereotyping and identifying those who live on council estates. Skeggs (1997, 2004) shows in her work that working-class women in particular are subjects of ridicule and prurient fascination, often sexualized, and associated with dirt and disease. The contemporary representations of ridicule relating to working-class women, and especially council estate mothers, relate to the wearing of tracksuits and gold jewellery, and having mixed-race babies; such portrayals are common within British television soap operas and comedy shows (e.g. Vicky Pollard in *Little Britain*, Bianca Butcher in *EastEnders*, Chantelle Garvey in *Benidorm*). These types of cultural references can invoke signifiers that do a great deal of work in coding a way of life that has been deemed valueless, and become more poignant when we are discussing working-class women whose bodies, appearance, bearing and adornment are also central in coding working-class people. When those symbols are connected to living space – and in particular the term 'council estate' – it leaves the reader or the viewer to 'join up the dots of pathologisation' in order to see and understand the picture: that certain ways of dressing, speaking and also where you live indicate a despised 'class position but also an underlying pathology' (Skeggs 2004, p. 37).

These representations of white working-class women have been documented previously. Bev Skeggs (1997, pp. 76–81) argues that working-class women are known as 'un-respectable' and have to work hard in becoming respectable, usually through adopting middle-class practices and by 'dis-identifying' from being working class. Chris Haylett (2001, pp. 360–63) further argues that to be 'white and working class' has become increasingly coded as 'backward' and un-modern. When negative representations of groups in society are commonplace, it has an effect upon how those groups are understood and also how they understand themselves (Skeggs 1997; Haylett 2000, 2001; Skeggs 2004; Welshman 2006; Lawler 2008). The women who live on the St Ann's estate in Nottingham know what 'others' think of them and a common theme in their interviews is the notion of being demeaned, 'looked down on' and made to 'feel small', as discussed in the next section.

Being looked down on

The women had an acute understanding of how they were known and 'looked down on' in wider Nottingham more widely and society generally because they lived on a council estate. They never denied where they thought they were positioned, often saying we are 'at the bottom' or 'lower class'. Yet they never tried to identify with 'middle class culture' in order to become 'respectable', instead finding value for themselves and their children from within the community, and through engaging in a local culture that they described as 'being St Ann's'. This was a local identity that was valued and had meaning for the women within the estate, but was not necessarily a valued identity that might be universally understood, such as the middle class, educated and respectable identity that Bev Skeggs (1997) notes.

The women discussed at great length the ways that they were represented in the media. For example, Tanya, a twenty-seven-year-old mother with three children under the age of five, explained that she could not understand why when a woman was supposed to be 'common' 'on the telly' (Matt Lucas's Vicky Pollard, Catherine Tate's Lauren, and Bianca from *EastEnders* were mentioned), they wore big hooped gold earrings, which she liked and which she thought suited her. Zena, another mother living on the estate with her two-year-old son and twelve-year-old daughter, told me that she 'knew' that some people would call her a chav not only because she liked wearing a lot of gold jewellery, but also because of the ethnicity of her children: 'too much gold, tracksuit and trainers, black baby in the pram.'

Gina was twenty-one, pregnant and lived alone with her six-month-old and two-year-old sons, who she described as 'quarter caste' – their father was mixed-race and lived on the estate with his mother, who was also involved in this research. Gina was one of many of the mothers who told me that she felt an acute stigma, particularly whenever she went to any of the benefit agencies. Although Gina was studying at a local college, she claimed income support and housing benefit and therefore was in constant contact with 'officials'. Gina told me that every time she gave her address to any of the 'officials' there was often a silence as they mentally processed her single-parent status, the ethnicity of her children, and then her address in St Ann's: 'I know what they're thinking you can see it ticking over in their brain as you wait for them to think "oh it's one of them from there".' Although negative social assumptions relating to lone mothers or mothers who live on council estates have been noted previously (Skeggs 1997; Gillies 2007), the women in St Ann's are particularly sensitive not only to the negative assumptions relating to being a lone mother living on a council estate, but also and in particular to being a white mother to mixed-race children. All of the women talked to me about how they were often sexualized because their children were signifiers and ultimate proof that they had sexual relationships with black men. Zena said to me that everyone thinks 'she's up for it', and Lynn, a woman in her forties with an adult daughter, described as being known as 'rough' because she came from a council estate, and also 'ready', meaning sexually available.

The women described their feelings of 'being looked down on', usually through their contact with 'others' who did not live on the estate. They also recognized the many aspects of their lives that stigmatized them. Mandy had lived in St Ann's with her own family her whole life and now she was in her mid-thirties and a mother living with her three sons on the estate. Mandy's middle son is autistic and she was advised by a social worker to go to the Gingerbread club, a local group of Nottingham mothers who met up with their disabled children. Mandy felt awkward when she arrived because the women there were 'not like' her:

> well I thought the people were posh people do you know what I mean the way they looked at me I felt really small I had to come out and my kids were playing up basically but I felt they were looking at me cos I was white and they [my kids] were mixed- race . . . no one talked to me yeah I felt that if I had said well . . . if they had said where are you from and I'd had said I'm from St Ann's they would have said oh yeah I can see why, that is how I felt . . . I wont there very long at all they dint mek me feel welcome. That Gingerbread club has been around for years I don't know if it's still going and I think that was one of the things that made me feel more secluded with my disabled son cos I felt like people were looking at me all the time at that Gingerbread club there was a lot of people there with disabled children do you know what I mean but they seemed posh and I felt that I was lower class.

Mandy was only one of the many women who told me about their experiences of feeling stigmatized and 'looked down on'. As a result of these feelings, they were extremely reluctant to meet anyone who they thought might be 'posh' or who might not understand their lives and, consequently, demean them. The women in St Ann's did not talk about engaging in a 'respectable performance' through the use of middle-class culture as Skeggs (1997, p. 94) notes; rather, they focused on resources of value, from what was available to them locally. This meant that some of the heavily stereotyped and negative aspects about 'being St Ann's' were celebrated by the women. All of them challenged the 'others' who looked down on them, stating that 'they could not live one day in our lives'. Furthermore, they also took pride in the fact that they 'badded it out' (coped with life's difficulties) on the estate, finding a sense of pride from overcoming the difficulties that they experienced. The women whom I met faced the challenges of living on the estate – and because of this, valuing 'being St Ann's', meeting those challenges, and dealing with the difficulties that the estate brought allowed the women to talk proudly about their daily lives. Therefore, it is important to understand what 'being St Ann's' means, as it is an identity that has recognized value within the neighbourhood and to the women. Using Pierre Bourdieu's (1977) system of capital exchange and value explains what happens in a community or within a group when there is a lack of status and respect, and community characteristics are developed under strain by local communities in order to compensate for the de-valuing of the neighbourhood and its residents in the form of an alternative value system. In 2013, 'belonging' and staying in St Ann's are important; consequently, the neighbourhood has strong meaning to those who live in it and being known and recognized in the community is very important. It may seem paradoxical that the residents who are stigmatized because they are known as living in St Ann's often described themselves as 'being St Ann's'. It is hardly surprising that if there are groups who are stigmatized and feel unwanted or of no value to the rest of society, they will find value for themselves, families and locality in what is available to them. This can be described as local social capital. The local networks, values and practices of the residents who live in St Ann's have a use value to them, although there is no exchange value on the outside of the estate. It may be the case that poor neighbourhoods have strong systems, resources and social capital but these are not recognized because they have no relationships with the institutional capital that can be exchanged in wider society, such as employment, as a route to becoming 'respectable'. As Ruth Levitas (2005 p. 168) argues, the fruitfulness of local social capital is often ruined because those resources are seen only as a means to an end and not as resources within themselves. Consequently, 'being St Ann's' and being valued locally were sources of both value and pride, attributes that the women described as being denied to them within wider society.

'Being St Ann's': the 'Jamaicanization' of a neighbourhood

'Being St Ann's' was the way that most women I spoke to described themselves. 'I'm typical St Ann's' or 'when you're St Ann's' was how the women often started a conversation. Being connected to the neighbourhood was extremely important: in order to show that they were St Ann's, the women described in great detail their family connections, the length of time they had lived in the neighbourhood and the depth of local knowledge they held about the area and its residents. This network and engagement located in the neighbourhood culture also meant that they could easily be recognized through ways of dressing and speaking, as well as through their 'taste' in music, food and social events. As noted above, most of the women wore a lot of gold jewellery, such as big creole earrings; some had gold-capped teeth; and expensive and branded sportswear and trainers were important for themselves and their children. These were ways that the women could show that they belonged to the estate; they knew what was valued and ensured that their children were also valued. The women discussed the ways and methods that they might save or earn money in order to buy expensive and designer-label clothes for their children. Birthday parties and christenings were also very popular on the estate and were events where the women 'showed off' their children. These gatherings were lavish affairs with expensive birthday cakes and gifts of jewellery, as well as new and extensively planned outfits for mothers and children.

'Being St Ann's' was also related to how they spoke in addition to how they looked and dressed. There is a distinct St Ann's dialect – a mixture of the local Nottingham accent interspersed with Jamaican words and speech patterns – which was described by some of the women as the 'street' language of St Ann's. I met two sisters, 'Kirsty' and 'Lucy', who were in their late teens and both of whose 'baby fathers' (a term used by the West Indian community meaning a child's biological father) came from Jamaica. They had lived on the estate since leaving Glasgow with their parents as very young children:

> Lucy: People has said to me "you think you're black cos you talk like that" well actually no I don't, I see it as street even now I'd get it as a big woman [adult] in the pub you know people say why you speak like that and I'm well that's how I've always spoke.
> Kirsty: Well a lot of people have said that I think I'm black and I wanna be black but I don't see it like that I see it like it was the community I was brought up in you know if you stick a black person in a white community they're gonna grow up white and if you stick a white person in a black community they're obviously gonna have black ways about them.

Although the use of specific West Indian styles of speaking and dressing are valued on the estate, these are not the only sites of value relating to the West Indian community: the Jamaican families, in particular, are themselves valued within the community. Therefore, being a part of one of the Jamaican families holds considerable worth. Many of the women discussed this as being particularly significant to 'being St Ann's' and the value of this specific multicultural identity has been described by the women as a 'modern', urban identity. The women on the estate understood that to be white and working class has become a de-valued position over the last thirty years: cultureless, backward and un-modern (Haylett 2001, p. 333). They recognized this through valuing what they thought was 'black culture' in contrast to what they described as being 'white'. As Pierre Bourdieu (1986, pp. 14–19) argues, it is those with the most power who get to decide what cultural resources are tasteful regarding ways of dressing, personal styling, music, art, speaking and social pursuits; while the culture of the middle class is deemed legitimate and tasteful, it is the culture of the working class that is illegitimate and lacking in 'taste'. Lawler (2008) and Skeggs (2004) transport this argument further by exclaiming that the cultural practices of the working class are not only 'tasteless' but are also pathologized, coded as immoral, wrong and criminal, and lacking in everything that is needed to be a part of a civilized modern Britain.

Once you go black you never go back

The ways in which heavily stereotyped images of black masculinity centring on sexual potency, 'coolness', criminality and macho aggression have both emerged and infiltrated the British psyche in recent years, especially in relation to white working-class youth culture, have been well mapped by various scholars (Hebidge 1979, Hewitt 1986; Back 1996; Gilroy 2000). The valued understanding of 'blackness' and Jamaican culture in St Ann's is equated with such ideas about black West Indian masculinity and is recognized as extremely prestigious in and around the estate. As such, you do not necessarily have to be 'black' or male in order to benefit from its value, as this masculinity is strongly associated with a street and urban culture and is expressed through language, music, food and dress.

Les Back (1996, p. 184) notes that the histories and cultural politics of the Caribbean and black America have formed the raw materials for a creative process in which 'black culture is actively made and re-made'. Based on his research during the 1990s in South London, he argues that a constant process of 'fashioning and re-fashioning' is happening within distinct and particular urban social relations, creating a cultural hybridity (Back 1996, p. 184). St Ann's in Nottingham has all the elements in place for the creative processes that allow 'black culture to be re-made' in negotiation with white working-class residents (Back 1996, p. 184). This is an extremely interesting and relevant use of cultural hybridity that has emerged in St Ann's. It adds another dimension in understanding contemporary identities and theorizing possible fragmentation in white working-class understandings of themselves, especially within multicultural urban neighbourhoods. It is not only the white mothers of mixed-race children who engage in this hybrid and entwined culture of 'blackness' and 'working-classness' on this estate; such behaviour is widely understood and practised throughout the estate. Claire, a mother with a ten-year-old daughter who describes herself as 'a lifer in St Ann's', explained how this particular understanding of 'blackness' works in practice:

> You see these white guys trying to walk like black people and you think God it must take you all day to get across the street but you're prepared to do it to keep this image and they have this tough face and you think "you're not black".

This is only one of many observations by the women in this research of how 'blackness' is often demonstrated within the estate, especially by young white men who appear to have practised 'being authentic' within the community through the visual markers of ways of dressing, walking and speaking. In fact, many of the women struggled to explain their own 'feelings' of ethnicity and the impact that 'mixedness' had upon the estate and their own lives. Gina, who had previously complained about how she thought the agencies see her, then went on to discuss how she sees herself:

> I don't see myself as full white neither do my friends especially black friends I don't think they see me as white or a white person, they know I'm white but they look at you different you know cos you've got mixed-race kids.

Gina also extended this complexity to her personal relationships: 'yeah I have tried to go out with a white boy before but the white boys think they're black they've got gold teeth they've got the black image so you might as well go out with someone real.'

When Gina talks about 'someone real' she is talking about 'authenticity' on the estate, and what is real and authentic for Gina is the black male, who also holds the most value for her. She demonstrates this in this next extract, in talking about how she thinks about 'white men':

> It might seem horrible but you know I think boring old white pub man, and I think of my Dad who just plays football and I know black people play football you know but I just think like beer belly and how they dress and then black people it is different you know you can go to all these different dances different music, food and it's interesting.

It seems that the taking on of 'black traditions and style' has resulted in a radical reconfiguration of white working-class culture in multi-ethnic locales (Hewitt 1986; Back 1996). This has led Gilroy (2000) to suggest that 'Black culture has become a class culture...as two generations have appropriated it and discovered its seductive meaning for their own' (2000, p. 273). The women in St Ann's understand the value and worth of what Gilroy terms 'black culture' and have appropriated it into their own lives, and for their own use passing it down to their children. In their interviews, they discussed how 'mixing' their own white working-class culture with an African-Caribbean culture has created something in the community that is superior to what they called 'the old days', when everything was 'white and boring'. The women on this estate constantly spoke of the pride they have of being 'more than just white' and of their 'beautiful mixed-race children' along with their modern 'multicultural families'. They regarded this mixing as the positive side of their physical, social and class positions – which without exception they understood as being 'at the bottom'. It was this part of their lives that they were most proud of, and this was apparent in the way in which they spoke about their children, whom they saw as special and beautiful. Moreover, they thought that they had given their children something that they and the estate valued: a birth status 'of not being just white'.

All of the women discussed how important this sharing of culture had been and the impact that it had made on their lives. Della, who was thirty-eight and raising her five children alone, told me that being part of the black British and Jamaican community in St Ann's and engaging in the culture connected with this community was extremely important for her. This was not just because she had mixed-race children:

> I've never really mixed with white people to me to go to a white club to me I don't feel like I fit in, if I go to a black club I feel more comfortable because that's the kind of music I like...I was into it even before I met the kids' Dad...I always mixed with black people so as I say for me to go to a white club I can't go to it cos I'm not into that sort of music I feel like the people aren't the same as me even though they're the same colour as me...you know people will say to me do you know you're white I know I'm white but it's hard to explain to someone who don't get it.

Lorraine, also in her thirties, was another single mother with five children and, like many of the mothers, had lived on the estate for most of her life and felt that she had a connection with the Jamaican community. Lorraine's family had moved into the estate in the early 1970s when they first arrived in Nottingham from Ireland. She was proud of her connection with the Jamaican community in St Ann's and talked about her childhood memories of dancing to reggae music and eating Jamaican food. Now Lorraine has her own children, she feels that it is important to cook Jamaican food at home. She also told me that there is a value attached to how authentically you can make Jamaican food, which is part of a wider value system of knowledge about Jamaican culture. Lorraine told me that anyone can cook chicken, but asked how many women her age, white or black, can cook good green banana:

> Well I think Irish and black mix really well they just do back in the day what was it no blacks, no dogs, no Irish what can you say...my auntie always went out with black guys so I used to go round there and she used to cook and the music was there so I was into it from about 10...I like the reggae music and the Jamaican food true dat I only listen to bare reggae music now and every day I have to cook bare food I have to cook curries, rice, Yam, green banana I have to cook everything how much white woman can cook all dem tings?

Appropriating the local culture, and engaging in the local value system through dress, food and speech, as Butler (1990) argues, is a matter of embodied social practice, a constant reiteration and 'performance' of particular discourses. The particular discourse here is of people who have become known as 'socially excluded' outside of the norms of society. Haylett (2001, p. 353) and Skeggs (2004, p. 111) argue that there has been a racialization of a specific group of white working-class people as 'the dirty white'. This group understand who they are and their own social positions through how they are judged and stigmatized in the media and wider social discourse. On this basis, it becomes all the more important for the women living in St Ann's to 'feel comfortable and fit in' within the estate that, simultaneously, allows them to be easily recognized on the outside.

Pride in mixed Britain

This connection to what the women on the estate know as 'black culture' and to the 'black community' is important to them as it is through this engagement that they feel like people of value on the estate. Nevertheless, there is often another aspect to this connection. When the women spoke of the things they liked about St Ann's, the area's multiculturalism was something they often brought up. Sharon, a woman in her fifties, has eight children, of whom the eldest six are white with mixed-race children – including Tanya, discussed earlier – and the two youngest are mixed-race. In talking of all the things they liked about St Ann's, Tanya and Sharon highlighted the local schools. Like many of the women, they held the primary schools in high regard and told me that they believe their children are gaining something really important by going to school in St Ann's. The 'multiculturalism' of the schools was often brought up as the extra value that their children were gaining:

Tanya: That's one of the positive things about St Ann's for the fact is that if you go to certain areas where the kids are all white then them kids have a thing there like a barrier with them people...cos they haven't mixed with them when they've mixed and they're all multi-cultural and they have had to learn things and then even in the classrooms here in St Ann's the teachers teach them what comes from the Chinese people and whatever else there is round here and that's good our kids don't grow up ignorant they know about multi-cultural things and that's good.

Sharon: I think that Sycamore is a good school they do loads of things for multi-cultural things...yeah they need to know about all different cultures the white and the black culture that's what I think is important both.

Tanya: I believe that there should be more multi-cultural teaching cos it's alright having them all together and them not learning from each other I think it should be a topic at all schools like Art, Maths and English yes because this is a multi-cultural country now.

Sharon: Well I think that eventually this country will be mixed race cos there's that many black and white people going together there's a lot of mixed race cos it's not the richer ones that are mixing it's us the lower ones so maybe our class will not be white anymore we will end up mixed race well that means that life's more interesting for us cos life was boring when I was young I've found out that it's more interesting being with a black man put it this way I've done more since I've been with them and I've learnt more and seen more than when I was with a white man.

Although it has often been argued that multiculturalism is a vague and confused concept having different meanings to different people (Modood 2004), the people in St Ann's explained their relationships, families and community as multicultural, and understood it as a sharing of culture, 'mixing it up'. The women often used the Jamaican national statement of 'out of many comes one people' as a way to explain what St Ann's has within its boundaries, and how it should be viewed. One community, many differences, but ultimately 'being St Ann's' and having this shared understanding is important.

Sharon's personal understanding of multiculturalism and mixedness has a much wider relevance. She describes herself as white and working class; she worked in the textile factories in Nottingham before de-industrialization hit the city. Sharon had six children from her previous relationship with her white working-class husband. However, she told me that being with her black partner meant that life was more 'interesting' now and had given her a value within the estate that she had not experienced previously: 'You used to go to parties and there was boring food but now it's all different food different music yeah I am proud of my mixed relationship.' Like all of the women on the estate, Sharon was extremely proud of her mixed-race family, and the thought of the white working-class no longer being white was not a worrying prospect for her; in fact, many of the women on the estate thought that all this mixing 'is good for us'. The white women who live on this estate with their mixed-race children and multiethnic families have creatively claimed value for themselves, and their lives, in contrast to and against what they understand is 'known about them' in wider society as poor, white working-class women.

Conclusion

This paper has introduced the narratives of the women living on the St Ann's estate. They speak candidly of the stigmatization that they feel, and the anger and pain that this causes, yet, despite this they find respect and pride for themselves and their children locally on this stigmatized council estate in Nottingham. The women have very little of the institutional capital that Bourdieu (1986) says is needed to be a person of value: they have limited formal education; those who work tend to be in unskilled and low-paid jobs; and they and their families live on a council estate. Their narratives tell that being valued and respected is important here as it is in any group in society. However, the women also tell of the pain and humiliation of been socially rejected by those on the 'outside'; they compensate by focusing and investing in what is local and available. This local practice forms an autonomous entity that is defined by a negative polarization to the norms of wider society and creates an alternative value system. By creating an alternative value system, those who are marginalized can create feelings of worth, power and status on the inside of their neighbourhood and among those who recognize and take part in the alternative value system (Cohen 2002, p. 28). Due to the complex nature of the estate, the alternative value system, and the elements that make up this system, are difficult to pin down. But the system also takes different forms for different groups within the estate. For women, a high value is placed on motherhood and therefore being a mother ranks highly on the estate. Indeed, being a mother and coping with the difficulties of living on the estate are often the only things that the women cite as being proud of in their lives.

There is a real and acknowledged pride in engaging in the local culture, which has been heavily influenced by black Jamaican culture, particularly for the mothers who have mixed-race children. Being authentic to the neighbourhood, being known and fitting in are other elements in becoming a person of value on the estate, but also to whom you are connected and how you are connected to the estate is equally important. In particular, there has been an exchange of culture on this estate: the women who live here are extremely proud of their success in 'mixing'. While this type of 'cultural mixing' has often been associated with 'youth culture', in St Ann's in Nottingham it is not limited to young people: it has become a hybrid and interchangeable culture that has grown throughout the whole community over a fifty-year period of the West Indian and white working-class communities living side by side.

Other literature relating to mixed families has highlighted and brought attention to the difficulties of interracial relationships and mixed identities. Vicki Harman's (2010) study and Ravinder Barn's (1999) work relating to social work practice highlight how white mothers with mixed-race children are often isolated and subject to racism with little support, thus urging professionals to consider the specific difficulties that mixed families encounter. Meanwhile, France Winddance Twine's (2010, p. 880) study of mixed families in the UK focuses on how white parents of whom she calls 'children of black Caribbean ancestry' negotiate racism and teach their children 'racial literacy' through engaging in black cultural forms.

This study in Nottingham recognizes the difficulties – and the women do not shy away from recounting their narratives of where and when they have experienced racism, and have struggled. However, they are resilient and have found ways of 'managing' through their use of the local support systems that can have huge benefits for families living on the estate, as well as penalties for the mothers in wider society. The women in St Ann's also value the Jamaican community and engage and invest in Jamaican culture, through food, music, clothing and ways of speaking. Twine also noted that white parents with mixed-race children invest in black cultural forms, but as ways of teaching their children how to cope with racism and their blackness. The women in St Ann's do not invest in these cultural forms as ways of teaching racial literacy to their children, but because it has a value on the estate and adds value to the women who have become devalued by the intersectionality between their whiteness and working-classness. This picture of modern Britain is complex. It shows how identity and community are closely linked, especially in stigmatized working-class neighbourhoods. The dynamic nature of multicultural Britain, and how racial identities are much more fluid than one may imagine, means that mothering across racialized boundaries on this estate is highly valued. It offers status and an opportunity to be more than a working-class white woman alongside a chance to engage in a contemporary multicultural Britain that in many other ways excludes and stigmatizes this group of women.

References

BACK, L. 1996 *New Ethnicities and Urban Culture: Racisms and Multi-Culture in Young Lives*, London: Routledge

BOURDIEU, P. 1977 *Outline of a Theory of Practice* (p. 192), Cambridge: Cambridge University Press, p. 192

———— 1986 *Distinction: A critique of the social judgement of taste*, London: Routledge

———— 1990 *The logic of practice*, Cambridge: Polity Press

BOURDIEU, P., *et al.* 1999 *The Weight of the World; Social Suffering in Contemporary Society*, Cambridge: Polity Press

BUTLER, J. 1990 *Gender Trouble*, London: Routledge

COATES, K. and SILBURN, R. 1970 *Poverty: The Forgotten Englishman*, London: Penguin Books

———— 1980 *Beyond the Bulldozer*, Nottingham: University of Nottingham

COHEN, S. 2002 *Folk Devils and Moral Panics: 30th Anniversary Edition: Creation of Mods and Rockers*, London: Routledge

DUNCAN-SMITH, I. 2008 Broken ghettos, *The Times*, 30 November, pp. 1–2

GILLIES, V. 2007 *Marginalised Mothers: Exploring working class experiences of parenting*, London: Routledge

GILROY, P. 2000 *There Ain't Black in the Union Jack*, London: Routledge

HARMAN, V. 2010 'Social work practice and lone mothers of mixed-parentage children', *British Journal of Social Work*, vol. 40, no. 2, pp. 391–406

HAYLETT, C. 2000 'Modernisation, welfare and "third way" politics: limits to theorising in "thirds"?', *Transactions of the Institute of British Geographers*, vol. 26, no. 1, pp. 43–56

———— 2001 'Illegitimate subjects? Abject whites, neo-liberal modernisation and middle class multiculturalism', *Environment and Planning D: Society and Space*, vol. 19, no. 3, pp. 351–70

HEBIDGE, D. 1979 *Subculture: The Meaning of Style*, London: Methuen

HEWITT, R. 1986 *White Talk, Black Talk: Inter-Racial Friendship and Communication amongst Adolescents*, Cambridge: Cambridge University Press

JOHNS, R. 2002 *St Ann's Nottingham: Inner City Voices*, Warwick: Plowright Press

LAWLER, S. 2003 *Rules of Engagement, Habitus, Power and Resistance in Feminism after Bourdieu*, Oxford: Blackwell Publishing

―――― 2005 'Disgusted subjects: the making of middle-class identities', *The Sociological Review*, vol. 53, no. 3, pp. 429–46

―――― 2008 *Identity: Sociological Perspectives*, Cambridge: Polity

LEVITAS, R. 2005 *The Inclusive Society*, 2nd edn, London: Macmillan

LISTER, R. 1996 *Charles Murray and the underclass: the developing debate commentaries*, London: IEA Health and Welfare Unit in association with The Sunday Times

MODOOD, T. 2004 'Capitals, ethnic identity and educational qualifications', in T. Bennett and M. Savage (eds), *Cultural Capital and Social Exclusion*, vol. 13 (2), No. 50, pp. 87–105, Basingstoke: Routledge

MUNT, S. (ed.) 2000 *Cultural Studies and the Working Class: Subject to Change*, London: Cassell

NAYAK, A. 2006 'Displaced masculinities: chavs, youth and class in the post-industrial city', *Sociology*, vol. 40, no. 5, pp. 813–31

―――― 2009 'Beyond the pale: chavs youth and social class', in K. Sveinsson (ed.), *Who Cares about the White Working Class*, Runnymead Trust

ONS (OFFICE FOR NATIONAL STATISTICS) 2007 *The English Indices of Deprivation 2007*, London: HMSO Communities and Local Government Publication

REAY, D. 2004 'Gendering Bourdieu's concept of capitals?: emotional capital, women and social class', in L. Adkins and B. Skeggs (eds), *Feminism after Bourdieu*, Oxford: Blackwell

REAY, D. and LUCEY, H. 2000 '"I don't really like it here but I don't want to be anywhere else": children and inner city council estates', *Antipode*, vol. 32, no. 4, pp. 410–28

RIDDELL, P. 2010 'We're living in broken Britain, say most voters', *The Times*, 9 February, pp. 9–10

ROGALY, B. and TAYLOR, B. 2009 *Moving Histories of Class and Community*, London: Palgrave Macmillan

SIBLEY, D. 1995 *Geographies of Exclusion: Society and Difference in the West*, London, London: Routledge

SKEGGS, B. 1997 *Formations of Class and Gender*, London: Routledge

―――― 2004 *Class Self and Culture*, London: Routledge

―――― 2009 'Haunted by the spectre of judgment: respectability value and affect in class relations', in K. Sveinsson (ed.), *Who Cares about the White Working Class*, Runnymead Trust

SOLOMOS, J. 2003 *Race and Racism in Britain third edition*, Hampshire: Palgrave

TWINE, F. W. 2010 *A White Side of Black Britain: The Concept of Racial Literacy*, Durham, NC: Duke University Press

WELSHMAN, J. 2006 *Underclass: A History of the Excluded 1880–2000*, London: Hambledon Continuum

WEST, E. 2009 'How to create an underclass: stalk council estates handing out condoms', *The Telegraph*, 14 August, p. 18

Index

Related titles from Routledge

Accounting for Ethnic and Racial Diversity

The Challenge of Enumeration

Edited by Patrick Simon, and Victor Piché

By the end of the 20th century, the ethnic question had resurfaced in public debate. Every country had been affected by what is commonly known as cultural pluralism, as a result of conflicts interpreted from an ethnic perspective.

This volume explores the ethnic and racial classification in official statistics as a reflection of the representations of population, and as an interpretation of social dynamics through a different lens. Spanning all continents, a wide range of international authors discuss how ethnic and racial classifications are built, their (lack of) accuracy and their contribution to the representation of ethnic and racial diversity of multicultural societies.

This book was originally published as a special issue of *Ethnic and Racial Studies*.

March 2013: 234 x 156: 156pp
Hb: 978-0-415-63113-6
£85 / $145

Ethnic and Racial Studies

Diasporas, Cultures and Identities

Edited by Martin Bulmer and John Solomos

This book comprises original research papers concerned with the role of diasporic ties and the social, cultural and political processes that are engendered by the changing experiences of these communities. Chapters cover a range of geopolitical and empirical contexts and serve to highlight the diverse theoretical and empirical questions that have become an integral part of the study of race and ethnicity in the contemporary environment. Although the role of diasporic communities has been the subject of historical reflection for some time, it is only now that the concept of diaspora has become a core theme in the social sciences and humanities. We have seen an ongoing discussion about notions such as diaspora, transnationalism and cosmopolitanism and their appropriateness as conceptual frames of reference for analyzing the diverse experiences of communities that have become dispersed across the globe. This collection makes an important contribution to this body of scholarship and research.

Diasporas, Cultures and Identities was originally published as a special issue of the journal *Ethnic and Racial Studies*.

December 2011: 234 x 156: 208pp
Hb: 978-0-415-68635-8
£85 / $145